ADVANCE PRAISE

"Andrew is living an inspired mission, educating men on such an important topic. His teachings are leaving a vast impact on humanity, and he will definitely leave a significant impact on your life."

—Dr. John Demartini, Human Behavioral Expert, Researcher, Author, Global Educator, and Founder of The Breakthrough Experience.

"I overcame my premature ejaculation and all my performance issues. Women now brag to all their friends about how I f*ck them and how long I last."

—James, Marketing Agency Owner

"I gained back my sex drive and libido. After working with Andrew, my wife felt like she was cheating with a different man. She said, 'Honey, we're back like we used to be, but better!'"

—Caleb, Business Owner

"Thanks to Andrew, I overcame my erectile dysfunction, porn addiction, and performance problems. Not to mention I've now found an amazing woman, and we have the most incredible connection inside and outside the bedroom."

—**Adrian,** Executive Engineer

"We're having a baby thanks to the work you did with my husband. I'm totally satisfied. He can't keep his hands off me, and now I'm pregnant! I don't know what you did to him, but thank you!"

—**Donna,** Business Coach and Mom

"I now can make every woman squirt, give any woman multiple orgasms, and make women scream so loud the neighbors know my name!"

—**Gun Hudson,** Entrepreneur and Investor

"I can love again. Before knowing Andrew, the love of my life died when I was fifteen (I'm now forty-one). I wasn't able to love fully until working with Andrew. After working with Andrew, I found a new love. We connect deeply, and we now have a kid on the way. Thank you!"

—**Ryko,** Artist

"I didn't feel like a man. I felt shut down and alone. I felt like no one understood me. I couldn't open up or ask for help. I felt trapped. Andrew helped me open up, connect deeply with my wife, and become a better dad to my two kids. I can't thank you enough."

—**Brett,** International Mining Manager

ANDREW MIOCH

BEST SHE EVER HAD

PRACTICAL ADVICE AND POWERFUL
TECHNIQUES SO YOU'RE THE ONE
SHE BRAGS ABOUT

To all the men who feel like there's no one to talk to about their sex lives, who want to feel deeply confident and share incredible experiences with women they care about.

To all the women who don't feel satisfied in their sex lives, and who dream of meeting men with the courage and confidence to be the best they ever had.

This book is for you.

DISCLAIMER

Some of the names in this book have been changed to protect the innocent (and the guilty). Over ten years of incredible sexual exploration, I've been fortunate enough to have many amazing experiences, some of which have been quite similar. If you're reading this book thinking you recognize yourself, think again.

CONTENTS

BEST SHE EVER HAD

Practical Advice and Powerful Techniques So You're the One She Brags About

ISBN   978-1-5445-2068-1   *Hardcover*

       978-1-5445-2067-4   *Paperback*

       978-1-5445-2066-7   *Ebook*

       978-1-5445-2069-8   *Audiobook*

INTRODUCTION

"Andrew, I fucking hate you."

I was halfway up a mountain when I got James's voicemail. I have no idea how I even had a signal.

"I don't even do business anymore. All I do is have sex with amazing chicks. It's all your fault. It's the middle of the day right now and I'm running around looking for different sex toys."

He was joking about hating me, of course. It's a running gag between us. Business and financial success have always been incredibly important to James. He never thought he'd be running around Melbourne in the middle of the week looking for sex toys. But since he transformed his sex life, he has been enjoying the incredible experiences he's been having.

When I met James, he was trapped in a nice-guy persona he'd been carrying around since childhood. Although he was highly successful in business, women walked all over him. He didn't know how to speak his mind or stand up for himself,

1

and the sexual experiences he craved seemed out of reach. In the business world, he was a boss, but his leadership skills didn't quite translate to the bedroom.

We connected through a mutual friend—a woman who recommended him for his copywriting skills. I saw a lot of myself in him and we chatted outside of work. Soon, we became friends. He helped me discover my authentic voice; instead of trying too hard to present myself as a slick, academic sexual educator, he encouraged me to express my true rawness. "You're not like that, man," he told me. "You're straightforward, no-bullshit. Show people who you really are."

My whole life has been about women, dating, and sexuality. James's whole life has been about business. I told him stories about some of my wildest nights, and he casually chatted about friends of his who were making $100,000 or more per month. I opened James's mind to what's possible sexually, and he did the same for me in business. One time, we were walking down Barkley Street in Melbourne and I started chatting to a cute waitress. Before long, I had a threesome lined up with her and my girlfriend. James couldn't believe it. In the same way, I went to parties with him where he introduced me to people who were killing it in business.

Before long, he started opening up to me about his struggles with premature ejaculation. He was putting too much pressure on himself to perform, and his cock was rebelling. I met with him and a girl he was seeing. She told me what was going on from her perspective—James was shy and nervous in the bedroom, cumming too quickly. She was losing respect for him as a man and her interest in having sex with him was declining.

Credit to James for sitting through that session while she went to town on his sexual shortcomings. It was incredibly painful for him to hear. But it was also the start of his determination to change. I could see that the feedback she gave him shook him to the core. I suggested that he come to one of my retreats, but he was already so wounded from the session he had with the girl he was seeing, he initially resisted. In reality, his confidence was at rock bottom. He was struggling to pick his self-worth up from the ground.

James's perception of his reality was so strong that he was fixated on it, to the point where he found it impossible to imagine something different. That led to a confrontation. James opened up about the fact that he felt like shit because he thought that, by his age, he should be better in bed. Understandably, he was scared to change. Shit got real, we had a heated discussion, and—despite his lingering skepticism— he ended up committing to the retreat.

That's when he turned a corner. He showed up on the retreat and decided, "Fuck it, I'm going to give it my all."

I get guys to do some weird shit on retreats. One of my favorite exercises is to make the shape of a pussy with my fingers and ask them to show me how they finger a woman. When James's turn came around, he was a little shy. I started giving him shit. "What the fuck was that?!" I asked.

3

He started laughing and his laughter soon spread through the other guys at the retreat. "Well, how am I meant to know this stuff?" he responded once his laughter subsided. "I've never been taught! I feel like I've been walking blind my whole life."

The retreat resulted in a series of epiphanies. He learned some techniques, but more important, he learned how to let go and flow in the bedroom. He got comfortable being dominant and expressing himself, both in a primal way and a slower, more gentle style. He stopped thinking that he had to *do* something and started to *feel*.

Two days after we wrapped the retreat, I got a call from James. Turns out he went out to a bar straight after the retreat finished and met a circus chick. They ended up going back to her place and fucking for five hours, from 11:00 p.m. until 4:00 a.m. She was doing crazy shit, like going into the splits. He pulled her hair, tossed her around, and transitioned into all sorts of different positions, while she encouraged him to pin her down and tie her up. For a man who was used to cumming in two minutes, this was revolutionary.

By the time they finished, this woman was convinced that he was a sex god. When he explained to her that, just a few days prior, he'd been clueless in bed, she loved his openness and vulnerability. James couldn't wait to speak to me. He left multiple missed calls on my phone and sent me a voicemail, saying, "I've never had a sexual experience like that. You've given me permission to explore aspects of myself I never dared to express before. I feel like I've unlocked myself, and I'm forever grateful."

Since that first retreat, James and I have worked together several times. Recently, we had a one-on-one session in which I shared some of the craziest shit I know with him, so he could take his sex life to the next level. This is a guy who, when we first met, was riddled with performance anxiety. Inside the bedroom, he had zero confidence and didn't feel like a man. Never in a million years did he think he would be where he is now, enjoying insane sexual experiences and lasting as long as he wants. James has as many women as he wants in his life, all of whom want more of him, because he's giving them the kind of pleasure they've never known with any other man.

The voicemail continued. "I hate you, but I love you at the same time. Now I can see what it's like to have truly great sex. I know what it is to connect deeply with myself and with women. And, even better, I have rock-solid self-respect and sexual confidence. My reality has totally shifted, and for that I want to send you a message of appreciation and gratitude, man. You've been such a blessing in my life."

SEXUAL PAIN IS AN EPIDEMIC

Maybe you picked up this book purely because you want to hear her scream your name—and you want the neighbors to hear, too. Let's face it, what man doesn't want to be the best she ever had?

But maybe there are deeper reasons. A lot of men are in pain. It may not be obvious, because it's not physical pain. It's the pain of feeling sexually broken or inadequate, or—in a milder form—like a sexual loser.

Sex and money are two of the hardest things to talk about. There are millions of people offering financial advice, but who can you turn to when you want advice on the most intimate parts of your life? According to the Cleveland Clinic, 52 percent of men in the United States suffer with erectile dysfunction (ED). Around 60 percent of the men I work with struggle with ED, premature ejaculation (PE), or both. Many of them have never discussed these problems with anyone before. If you're in their position, it's okay. The worst thing you can do is suffer in silence.

In modern society, we do a shitty job of sex education. Maybe you suffered through watching an embarrassed teacher put a condom on a banana when you were a teenager. It's better than nothing, but only just. When you had questions about sex or sexuality, who did you turn to? Was there anyone you felt you *could* turn to?

We've wasted too much time turning sex into a taboo subject. It's time to normalize talking about sex and let go of the pain that comes with dissatisfying, subpar sexual experiences. In the absence of real education, we get our sexual education from porn or banter with friends. But neither of these addresses our deepest insecurities.

Maybe you're worried about the size or shape of your cock. Maybe you struggle to get it up or keep it up, cum too early, or find it difficult to cum with a partner. Or maybe you just sense that there's more to sex, and long for a deeper connection.

Be honest with yourself: is there anything that matters more to you than the quality of your sex life? It doesn't matter how successful you are in other areas of your life. If you're unable to connect deeply with your wife, partner, or lover, it gnaws away at you, souring your experience of life.

Imagine you're with a beautiful woman, a new girlfriend. You're lying together in bed, gazing deep into each other's eyes. You've just had incredible sex, and in your heart, you're longing to tell her how much you care about her. But you can't seem to get the words out. No matter how hard you try, they stick in your throat. Something in your brain tells you that tenderness equals weakness, and you clam up.

You might get away with that the first time, but if it becomes a pattern, your woman will notice. If you can't express yourself fully, she'll feel that you're not truly with her, and she'll become dissatisfied. She may think you're not really into her. As the connection erodes, you'll probably be less turned on. The experience will feel lackluster and meaningless. You won't feel an emotional connection. Neither will she.

The distance between you grows and you look elsewhere for sexual satisfaction. She has a "headache" more and more often. Perhaps you start visiting brothels or take a side chick. Shit, maybe you start jerking off in your car, so you don't have to face her. Prostitutes, side chicks, and masturbation ease the ache, but all you really want to do is talk to your girlfriend. Of course, you don't. What would you tell her? Neither of you feel heard, understood, or appreciated. Gradually, you lose hope. It seems like you're in a downward spiral and you don't know how to reverse it.

You look for help in spiritual communities and kink/BDSM subcultures, but they seem too out there. Is getting naked in front of strangers really an essential part of improving your sex life? Are you sexually unfulfilled if you don't have a dungeon full of whips and chains? All you want is some relatable, concise sexuality advice, so that you can reconnect with your woman and start enjoying better, more pleasurable sex. The other stuff can come later.

If you visit a doctor, they give you the dispiriting message that you're stuck with sexual dysfunction for life. Viagra gets you hard when you need to, but it doesn't fill the growing emotional void. Plus, you may experience long-term side effects, such as issues with heart function and blood pressure. Even a sex therapist may not be able to help you. Their clinical, academic perception of reality has little in common with the messy reality. With a lack of good information—and an abundance of misinformation—you start to feel that you're completely on your own.

If you stay in a relationship, you're no longer lovers. At best, you're like roommates, friendly and polite but unable to express attraction and desire. At worst, you become bitter and resentful. Perhaps she cheats on you. Maybe you break up and the cycle starts again with a new woman. Instead of loving sex, you start to dread it. It's painful to keep putting yourself through disappointments.

It's time for all of that to change. That's why I wrote this book. My mission in life is to elevate the sexual well-being of humanity. My purpose on this planet is to support men in having mind-blowing sexual experiences with women they care about. I truly believe that every man deserves a proper sexual education. That's not merely about performance. It's also about honesty, vulnerability, and self-expression.

THE VISION OF
SEXUAL QUANTUM LEAP

The underlying purpose behind everything we do at Sexual Quantum Leap is this:

"To elevate the sexual well-being of humanity, so men can have mind-blowing sexual experiences with women they care about, by opening their hearts and connecting deeply with themselves. As a result, they become the best she's ever had, both inside and outside the bedroom."

I've been through the same shit you've been through. I've experienced erectile dysfunction and premature ejaculation. I've struggled to get it up and seen the look of disappointment on a woman's face. I know what it's like to lie in bed thinking, "Come on, bro, it's go time," only for my cock to refuse to respond. I've sat in my car outside of a brothel, thinking, "Fuck, am I really gonna do this?" I felt so blocked, and the connection felt so far gone, that I didn't believe I could possibly resuscitate it. I didn't want to go behind my partner's back, but the relationship felt so stale and boring that I was desperate for some excitement. She wasn't doing what I wanted to do in the bedroom, and I didn't know how to communicate with her. It was a horrible situation. I loved her so much, but I felt trapped in a depressing situation that I didn't know how to change.

PERMISSION TO LOVE SEX

Sounds terrible, right? Unfortunately, this is the reality for millions of men. Perhaps it's close to your reality. If so, it doesn't have to be. James never imagined he could enjoy the sex life he does today. He might sometimes tell me he hates me, but mostly he's amazed by the quality and depth of his sexual connections.

Like James, so many men get stuck in their heads. They think sex is a specific sequence of moves, and that all they need to do is make the moves in the right order, and—bingo!—they'll be good in bed. But sex is a dance. It's a flow. The real pleasure comes from dropping into your body and accessing the physical sensations that make you and your woman feel so good. Before anything else, good sex starts with presence.

Sex is about sensation. It's fun, it's playful, it's messy. It's a process of curiosity and exploration. There's no one-size-fits-all road map I can give you that will guarantee good sex every time. That might seem like bad news, but it's actually *great* news. You don't need to be perfect. You don't need to give up on your desires and become totally focused on her pleasure. You get to explore, laugh, and discover.

If there's one thing I want you to take away from this book, it's permission to tap into and express your sexual desires, and to invite the woman you're with to express hers. You're not on your own here. Every chapter contains key insights, and most include practical exercises. But everything starts from the understanding that it's okay to be sexual. It's okay to want sex. When you and the woman you're with both feel heard and understood, you'll open the path to beautiful, raw, enriching sexual experiences for both of you.

Too many men—and women—deny themselves pleasure because they feel shame or guilt around their sexuality. The purpose of this book is to open you up to your full sexual potential, from tender caresses to wild, primal, animalistic fucking. From humor and playfulness to sobbing in each other's arms. From incredible peaks of pleasure to deep emotional connections. It's all possible and it's a lot more accessible than you probably realize.

The even better news is that you don't need to forego your own pleasure and think only about pleasuring your woman. I'm not suggesting that you behave selfishly, but I *am* saying that when you know your own body and understand what you want and like, you'll dramatically increase your attractiveness. Women can feel that level of presence, and they're naturally drawn to it. Authentic expression is sexier than holding back, any day of the week.

Deep sexual connection will flow from your comfort with your sexuality, and your capacity to put the woman you're with at ease. This book is dedicated to helping you find that, both through deep insights and through practical exercises you can do again and again, whenever you need to reconnect with your presence and your pleasure.

In Chapter One, You're Not Fucked Up, You're Not Broken, we'll discuss the incredibly common male fear of being sexually abnormal. Don't worry, you're not. Chapter Two, Six Sexual Mindsets, is about sexual personal development. It centers on the mindsets you'll want to bring to your interactions with women.

Chapter Three, Leadership Is Love, describes the power of holding a dominant frame. We'll discuss the difference between dominance and being domineering, and explain why dominance, exercised correctly, is a gift to women. Next up, in Chapter Four, Know What You Want, Ask for What You Want, we'll cover the power of understanding and acting on your desires.

Chapter Five is called Every Woman Is Different, Every Pussy Is Different. The central point of this chapter is that you need to connect with the woman in front of you. Techniques are great, but they're no substitute for genuine curiosity and care. Chapter Six, Practical Ways to Boost Your Sex Life, is packed with ideas you can explore with a partner.

Although this isn't a book about relationships, it would be incomplete without some discussion of what will inspire a woman to fall in love with you. Chapter Seven, Inside and Outside the Bedroom, fills this gap. Finally, Chapter Eight, Leave Her Better and Wetter, concentrates on a fundamental principle: always improve her life, whether you spend one night together or five decades.

If you read the entire book, you'll learn how to confidently ask for what you want in bed, and how to support yourself and your partner in living out your true sexual desires. We'll discuss how to bring up sex so that you both feel excited to talk about it, how to create thrilling date nights, and how to facilitate nights where one of you gets your every desire met.

You'll learn how to speak from the heart without becoming so woo-woo that you chop off your balls. How can you open up in the bedroom? How can you find the courage to express yourself verbally? How can you give yourself permission to say what you want to say? You'll also learn how to deepen your sexual connection with your partner. Many people believe that sex inevitably becomes stale over time. It doesn't have to. It can go in the opposite direction, as you and your partner understand one another more intimately.

Some men find that, as they fall more deeply in love with a partner, they struggle to express themselves sexually. They feel it's harder to be raw and uninhibited with the woman who might one day be the mother of their children. Again, this isn't inevitable. Your sex life can become deeper and wilder even as you fall more powerfully in love. That said, you don't have to restrict yourself to one woman. You can use the information in this book to explore your sexuality with multiple women, if that's what you desire.

As an additional bonus, I've scattered links to some of my best material throughout the book. Not everything is best expressed in writing. Some ideas come across better using audio or video. I've collected a huge range of cool shit at the following link: sexualquantumleap.com/resources.

This link isn't listed on the main website. The only way you can get there is by typing the URL directly into a web browser. As you read, you'll see this link mentioned several times, whenever we cover a subject with an additional training, or an audio or video bonus.

Okay, let's go. You've picked up this book, so you've already taken the first step toward creating an amazing sex life for yourself.

WHO IS ANDREW MIOCH?

You might be wondering why the hell you should listen to me. Who is this Andrew Mioch guy anyway, and what does he know about sex? Here's the Cliffs Notes version.

I've always been fascinated by the opposite sex. Way back in grade two, my teacher wrote on my school report that I got distracted by anything in a dress. "Fuck," said my dad. "I send you to a good Christian school and this is what happens." I guess my destiny was written in the stars. Over the years, my obsession has only gotten worse.

Fast-forward to my teens, and I was fascinated by all kinds of personal development material. In particular, I loved anything about female psychology, sexual psychology, or relationships. Everywhere I went, night or day, I took the opportunity to meet women. I made a lot of connections, although I also got rejected a ton along the way. Naturally, I thought I was great in bed. I couldn't have been more wrong.

I wasn't particularly academic; I was a tradie (Australian slang for a tradesman). To be specific, I worked as a carpenter. At the time, my vocabulary consisted of about four words. I had attended a few trainings on stepping up, being a man, and owning my desires, but none of them deeply hit home. When I finished school, I thought I was too dumb to go on to college or university, so I jumped into carpentry as a way to earn money.

In my mind, I was a real bad boy. I had three girlfriends, all of whom thought we were monogamous. I was fucking a married woman and—behind her back—one of her best friends. On top of all this, I was selling drugs, doing promotions at a nightclub, and hanging with criminal biker gangs. I thought the only way I could get what I wanted was by lying and cheating. It was a chaotic time.

Underneath the posturing, I was a scared kid in search of validation, love, and acceptance. Of course, I got caught, both by the women and by the cops. The women were seriously pissed off. The cops charged me with seven offenses. I thought I was going to jail. I was nervous as fuck. Fortunately, the judge took pity on me. Instead of sending me to jail, she gave me a hundred hours of community service.

One of my community service supervisors—the second-in-command—was a woman. She had recently broken up with her boyfriend and she invited me over to her house. I rode over on my motorbike, thinking she wanted a little emotional support. It never occurred to me that we'd fuck. Shows what I knew. She opened the door wearing a skimpy little outfit and we got straight to it.

This supervisor looked like a real Goody Two-Shoes, but behind the scenes dozens of guys were paying her for sex. Sometimes she had sex with seven or eight guys in a *day*, then met me later. I didn't know any of this until she told me. "Holy shit," I thought. "She's living a double life." At one point, I had a threesome with her and one of my best mates; she was doing shit that was out of this world.

Then one day, in bed, she dropped a bombshell. "You know what, Andrew?" she told me. "I'm going to be 100 percent honest with you."

"Okay," I replied.

"You're shit in bed," she continued. "I'm not enjoying this."

It was like a dagger to the heart.

With hindsight, what she was telling me should have been obvious. She was so good in bed that, in comparison, I didn't have a clue. When I calmed down, I realized I had two options. I could get pissed off and refuse to take responsibility, or I could use what she told me as a catalyst for learning everything I could about sex. I chose option B.

After I was told I was shit in bed, I figured I needed mentors to learn how to be better. I met my first mentor, Shae, and took his course twice. I willingly drove an hour—or, if traffic was bad, an hour and a half—to go to his house, sit with him for a few hours, and listen to him talk about sexuality and spirituality. Suddenly, I was in rooms full of people discussing the juncture between sexuality and spirituality, about creating deeper connections in the bedroom, about opening up and expressing emotions. I did crazy exercises aimed at releasing raw sexual expression. It was a whole new world to me. Most of the time I found myself thinking, "What the fuck is this?" Nonetheless, I was hooked!

Shae's an incredibly humble, loving man, with enormous knowledge about sexuality, Eastern philosophies, and human development. Through working with him, I started to discover that I could be both soft and raw in the bedroom. He opened my mind to new aspects of my masculinity and treated me like a son. Even today, we remain great friends. I still share some of the great material I learned from his course, The Way of the Black Dragon, and from our wide-ranging discussions about life and sexuality.

Shae also introduced me to the guy who would become my second mentor, Dom. "This guy's in Sydney," Shae told me. "You guys should link up."

Dom was the highest-paid dominant male in Sydney. He got paid a shitload of money to give women sexual experiences they would never forget. He was also a crazy motherfucker who had about 50 kilos (110 pounds) of sex toys at his house. Dom took me under his wing and introduced me to the kink scene. I'll never forget the first time he took me to an underground kink party. I was fucking terrified. He told me to wear all black and gave me a little whip to wield.

Dom wasn't a conventionally attractive guy, but he was always surrounded by hordes of women. As soon as I met him, it was clear he knew something powerful. He was a master of making women comfortable, allowing them to express themselves sexually. When we walked into the club for that first party, I vividly remember seeing someone hanging from the ceiling. "What the fuck is this?" I wondered. I got used to it quickly. A little later, we had two women bent over a pool table, screaming with pleasure as we whipped them.

Another night, Dom took me to a very underground club, where I saw women forming a queue waiting for him to give them an experience they would never forget—and he did. Sometimes he had seven to ten women waiting for their turn to have a sexual experience with him. Dom never disappointed, using his hands and toys to give women incredible pleasure. He regularly made women squirt, spraying a wildly applauding audience. I assisted him, pleasuring the women with a toy while he taught me what to say and do.

I spent around a year around Dom, an incredibly eye-opening time. I had never met someone so comfortable with his sexuality, and so skilled at giving women incredible experiences. The biggest lesson I learned from him, however, was an understanding of female sexual psychology. It was from Dom that I came to understand how kinky women can be, and that there are truly no limits in the realms of sexuality. When I stayed at his place, I saw and heard things that blew my mind.

Once I got used to the environment, I started striking out on my own. I read a bit, watched videos, took more courses, and attended some sex parties, swingers' parties, and kink events in Melbourne. That's where I met my next mentor, Red. Red has been active in the kink scene for decades and runs the biggest kink party in Melbourne. She taught me how to massage and eat a woman's pussy, how to give women multiple orgasms, and how to be dominant in the bedroom.

At first glance, you'd never guess that Red is a lynchpin in the kink scene. She's quirky and academic, with an alternative style that hints at hidden depths, without revealing the extent of her wildness. She's extremely humble and deeply loving, yet she models strong boundaries and knows exactly how to fulfill her needs and the needs of her partners.

My current mentor is an incredibly wise, grounded guy named Tao. He's one of the most loving people I've ever met, with nothing to prove and a huge desire to serve. Tao has found the sweet spot between conceptual education and direct, spiritual teaching, making his teachings very grounded in reality. He does an extraordinary job of bringing East and West together. Tao's depth of wisdom is second to none and I anticipate calling him a mentor for the rest of my life.

After immersing myself in a diverse range of sexual subcultures, I started running my own sex parties. By this time, my dating game was on point and I could meet women almost anywhere. It was easy to get them excited about coming to the parties. Usually, there were about thirty or so people attending, at a ratio of roughly two women for each man. It was wonderful to see how, in the right environment, the women who attended the parties allowed themselves to be fully sexually expressed.

One time at a party, I made four women in a row squirt. None of them had ever had that experience before. They didn't think it was possible for them. But within two minutes, all of them turned into waterfalls. As I pleasured two women at once, other guys watched us. "How the fuck did you do that?" one of them asked. "You have got to teach us." They couldn't believe that the women felt so safe, so connected, and so open after knowing me for such a short time.

The more I shared what I'd learned during my sexual apprenticeship, the more I saw how men were starving for practical, relatable advice on sexuality. I realized, too, that the men I met didn't just want meaningless physical pleasure. They craved deeper connections and genuine emotional fulfillment.

I traveled the world seeking out the best mentors and found that the same principles apply everywhere.

That's when I began to think about writing a book, to reach more men than I will ever meet in person. Sexual education is so needed right now. I'm still a student—Red told me that she still feels like a beginner after thirty-five years—but I've come a long way from the kid who was gobsmacked watching Dom make women scream with pleasure in front of hundreds of people at my first kink party. It's time for me to put my best material into print and do what I can to accelerate the sexual evolution of humanity.

WHAT YOU CAN—AND CAN'T—EXPECT FROM THIS BOOK

By the time you finish this book, I want you to feel sexually empowered. I want you to know that you can share incredible sexual experiences with women you care about, without relying on pills, sprays, and creams.

If you're invested in personal development, you probably think nothing of dropping a couple of grand on a new course that you trust will take you to the next level in your health or business. But do you invest the same amount in your sexuality? Most men don't. But why the hell not? We all know sex is super important. This book will fill that gap. It's a guide to your sexual personal development.

You can trust me to give it to you straight, with no bullshit. I might challenge your beliefs—I might even hurt your feelings—but it's all because I have your best interests at heart. Everything in these pages is tried and tested, by me and by the thousands of clients I've worked with from all over the world. I hope that you'll come to see me as a friend. Sure, I might give you a bit of tough love at times, but it's only because I want you to have the sexual experiences that I know you're capable of, and that you want for yourself.

While this book is a guide to sexuality, it's not a manual. You won't find any diagrams explaining where to find the clitoris or the G-spot. Nor is this book aimed at helping you tackle deep-seated sexual trauma. I'm not a sex therapist, sexologist, or doctor. I'm just a guy who wants you to consistently enjoy peak sexual experiences, and hear women tell you that you're the "best she ever had."

We'll touch on aspects of relationships, but this isn't a relationship book. When you're confident in your sexuality, you'll undoubtedly relate differently to women, and that will likely have a massively positive impact on your dating life. When you meet a chick knowing that you can give her a mind-blowing experience in the bedroom, you'll talk to her differently. You'll smile quietly to yourself and approach her with the inner confidence that can only come from knowing how to wield your weapon for maximum orgasmic potential. There's some crossover between sexuality and relationships. But, again, we don't tackle specific relationship issues here. Our real aim is for you to feel comfortable talking about sexuality, without an ounce of shame or guilt.

Importantly, this book isn't a quick fix. There's no magic bullet that will take away all your sexual challenges in the blink of an eye. I share tips and techniques, but I don't want you to rely solely on tips and techniques. Tips and techniques constitute about 10 percent of sexuality. Beyond that, you need to understand your own sexual psyche, and the sexual psyche of the woman in your life. If you want your sexual life to change, you'll need to absorb the lessons in these pages and do the work. Issues such as premature ejaculation and erectile dysfunction are relatively easy to resolve, but sexuality isn't a one-and-done scenario. The journey to deeper pleasure and connection is never-ending.

Finally, and this is completely nonnegotiable, this book is not for men who want to manipulate or coerce women. If that's where you're coming from, put this book down now and get some psychological help. But if you're a good man, who has women's best interests at heart, and want to share incredible sexual experiences with women you care about, keep reading.

CONSENT, CONSENT, CONSENT

This shouldn't need to be said, but in the age of #MeToo, unfortunately, it does. Everything in this book is intended for the benefit of consenting adults. Always, *always*, make sure that you have consent—and that your partner is legally an adult.

We're going to talk about some risky subjects, and there's absolutely nothing wrong with playing at your edges, and hers. But don't go beyond them. Use safe words. Get explicit consent if you need to. You might think you're killing the mood, but women will relax when they know you care enough about them to have honest, open conversations. That can only be good for both of you, and for the quality of your sexual connection.

1

YOU'RE NOT FUCKED UP, YOU'RE NOT BROKEN

It was 4:00 a.m. in Warsaw when Brandon called me. I'd had a big night and hadn't been to bed yet. As I picked up his call, I looked over the balcony of my hotel at the city unfolding below me.

Brandon knew me from Facebook and Instagram posts, and he was thinking of coming to one of my retreats. With the time difference—me in Poland, him in the United States—we fucked up the timing of the call and booked it for the middle of the night, my time.

He's an Asian guy with a strict family upbringing. Very smart and confident in most areas of his life, but a mess sexually. Growing up, he got some seriously damaging messages about his sexuality. Don't talk about sex. Repress all sexual desire. If necessary, learn from porn. And don't *ever* talk about sexual frustration. Not surprisingly, he had PE, ED, and a chronic shortage of women in his life.

Brandon's parents wanted their son to be perceived as a financial and social success, which would have made him acceptable in the eyes of their community. His sexual experience was less of a concern. His natural desire was getting totally squashed and he didn't know who to turn to for help. He felt trapped by his parents' restrictive views, living the life they had mapped out for him and unable to explore his sexuality like a normal college kid. He couldn't open up to women or to his college friends, who subscribed to the same ideas as his parents. He felt as though the only message he was getting about sex was that he needed to find a good Chinese wife and stay with her for the rest of his life.

Frustrated as he was by that expectation, he was also riddled with shame and guilt for wanting to go against it. He questioned whether *he* was at fault for being unable to live up to his parents' expectations. Was there something wrong with him? When he saw some of my videos, it clicked for him. Other people felt the same way about sexuality. He wasn't alone, and he wasn't some kind of freak.

Brandon's a smart guy with a gift for public speaking and debate, and he made a great case to me for jumping on a plane and going to an upcoming Sexual Quantum Leap retreat in Thailand. But then he backtracked and started arguing against himself, saying he couldn't afford it.

I asked him for permission to be 100 percent honest with him. He said yes, so I gave him both barrels. "What's the alternative?" I asked him. "You don't know how to connect sexually, you don't know how to open up, and your masturbation habits are fucked up because you've had so much of a guilt trip from your parents. I don't want you looking back at your life when you're seventy, regretting that you settled for an average woman and a lifetime of shitty sexual experiences. Do you really want to spend the rest of your days struggling with PE and ED, getting told you're fucked up, and relying on harmful pills to get hard?" The line went quiet for a moment. Then he said, "Fuck, you're right. I'll get back to you."

This conversation happened just a week before the retreat, but Brandon was as good as his word. He found the balls to confront his parents, telling them that he needed some real sexual education and that learning from porn was no substitute. Eventually, a couple of days before the retreat, they caved and agreed to pay for him to participate.

When Brandon walked into the retreat, he was nervous as hell. He could hardly believe he had made it. At the same time, he was a little skeptical. Could he really change radically in a few days? He gave me a hug and said, "Thank you for the opportunity. I'm fucking scared, but I'm going to be all in."

SEXUAL EDUCATION IS MISSING

Most men think they're fucked up and broken. Why? Because they've never received any competent sexual education.

What sexual education did you get when you were at school? A few embarrassing and hilarious sessions on anatomy? If you were at a religious school, you probably didn't even get that. You were just told not to have sex before marriage.

The less education you had, the more likely you are to be stuffed full of shame and confusion about your sexuality. And that energy has to go somewhere. When you suppress your sexuality, it usually gets expressed in unhealthy ways. Teen pregnancies and STDs, anyone? Yeah, those are one result of not giving teenagers the education they need to make sense of their sexual desires.

I've heard it said that, in any profession, 20 percent of the practitioners are phenomenal, 20 percent are quite good, and 60 percent are absolutely fucking terrible. If that's true, we're failing badly in the field of sexuality. Even some professionals don't know how to handle this shit.

I've spoken to doctors, sexologists, and sex therapists who don't have a clue how to talk to real people about sex. I've spoken to people who visited doctors for help and found that the doctors were embarrassed to say the words "penis" or "vagina." Many sexologists and sex therapists know how to talk conceptually about sex but get stuck in their heads, describing sex in an academic way that bears no relation to the messy, joyful reality.

How are people supposed to feel okay about discussing one of the most intimate parts of their lives with professionals who aren't comfortable with the vocabulary of their field of exper-tise? Many people who turn to doctors, sexologists, or sex therapists for help end up feeling even more alone. It's not the entire profession, by any stretch of the imagination, but it's enough for a significant proportion of people to feel like they're not getting the help and advice they need.

At the other end of the spectrum, the tantric sex scene is littered with people on a power trip, more interested in confirming their own identity as a sex god or goddess than on providing a genuine sexual education. A lot of events require participants to get naked straightaway and do things that they may be uncomfortable with, such as masturbate in a group of strangers or get anally fingered by another man. I speak from personal experience. Tantric sexual practices can be great, but not when they're an extension of the teacher's ego, based on bullshit and pseudoscience.

What happens? People don't know where to go for help. They conclude that they're fucked up and broken and retreat back into guilt and shame. Or they go the other way and do things they don't want to do. They may banter with their friends about sexuality, without revealing their true vulnerabilities or finding genuine answers. I've worked with thousands of men, many of whom have told me: "Thank God you do what you do. I've never told anyone this."

That's the gap I want this book to bridge. We're going to go through some practical shit that will help you become better and more comfortable in bed. The first thing to understand is that you are *not* fucked up and broken. It doesn't matter if you struggle to get it up sometimes, or if you tend to cum too quickly. It doesn't matter if you can't cum at all. It doesn't matter what size or shape your cock is. You're normal. You know how I know that? Because you're human.

If you're judging your manhood against a perceived scale of cock size and bedroom performance, you're putting a hell of a lot of pressure on yourself before you even get naked with a chick. If you're going into sexual relationships beating yourself up because you feel like you have to look and behave a certain way, of *course* you're going to struggle. I want to take the pressure off of you.

The true measure of a man is character, not cock size. How well can you express your emotions? How deeply can you connect with the woman in front of you? How honest and vulnerable do you dare to be?

If you have erectile dysfunction, that can be cured. If you have premature ejaculation, that can be cured. The solutions are surprisingly simple, and we'll cover them in a later chapter. You don't need to rely on a pharmaceutical industry that tells you you're broken and the only way to fix your problems is with a pill. Oh, and by the way, you'll be taking it for the rest of your life.

I personally know a guy—an international dating coach—who was told at the age of eighteen that, for the rest of his life, he would need Viagra to get hard. He believed the doctor who told him this and it has fucked up his life. The guy is now thirty-three years old. He still sometimes uses drugs and alcohol to suppress his feelings of unworthiness and feel normal. In my opinion, the doctor was guilty of malpractice. I'm not telling you that you shouldn't take a Viagra if you've got a big night planned and want to stay hard for hours, but if you feel like you *need* pharmaceuticals to function long-term, something has to change.

One of my main motivations for writing this book is because it's time for sex to stop being taboo. I want to raise the veil, so you feel comfortable exploring and expressing your sexuality. It's totally normal to want deep emotional, physical, and spiritual connection with women you care about. It's not fucked up at all to aspire to that. Quite the reverse. If you think you're broken, you'll likely stifle the connection, intimacy, and passion.

A lot of men get stuck either taking too much responsibility, or none at all. Either they think that "chicks are crazy" and refuse to acknowledge their part in things going off the rails, or they feel like their sexual challenges are entirely their own fault. The truth is that sexuality is a learnable skill, just like business, tennis, or piano. The only difference is that most of us have never had the opportunity to learn about sexuality!

YOUR SEXUAL STORY

We all have a sexual story. We create that story from all the sexual influences in our life: parents, friends, school, early experiences. We put all that information together and turn it into a narrative about who we are sexually. The problem is that many of us can't tell the difference between story and reality. We think that story is *who we are* sexually, and there's no way we can change it. That's not true.

31

Exercise:
Your Sexual Story

Before you read the rest of this book, I want you to go ahead and complete this simple yet profound exercise.

First, write the word "sex" on a piece of paper. Then, conduct a word association. Write whatever comes up, without self-censoring. Positive, negative, anything. Teenage anxieties, religious repression, peak experiences; get it all onto the page. You don't need to share it with anyone.

Second, write a letter to Sex. Start it "Dear Sex," and continue as though you were writing a letter to a person. "I feel like I've been neglecting you," for example. "I'm sorry I treated you badly." Whatever you want to say to Sex, put it on the page. Include the positive stuff, too. That amazing blow job in the car. Times you've felt massive appreciation of your sexuality.

Finally, write the story of the sexual man you see yourself becoming, in the present tense. "I go to sex parties," perhaps. "I know how to make women squirt." Or, "I have an amazing, loving partner and we have incredible, connected sex." Whatever you see yourself stepping into as a sexual man.

> Once you've done this, read your new sexual story to yourself in the mirror every day. If you want it to become real, you need to make it true. Before you can see it manifest in the physical world, you need to feel it in the metaphysical world.

We all pick up ideas about sex from the people around us. But those people have picked up ideas from *their* parents, teachers, and peers. How do we know what's really true for us, unless we take the time to examine our sexual story?

Your body is your own, and no one else gets to tell you how to enjoy it. As long as you're not hurting anyone, you're free to explore and find out what pleases you. This beautiful body is essentially just a pleasure station, but so many of us are trapped by beliefs about how and where and when it's okay to feel pleasure. Personally, I always feared that massaging my prostate was "gay," until a mentor encouraged me to give it a try, and I discovered that it feels amazing.

If you're going to fully express yourself sexually, it's essential that you understand your sexual story. Then, you can let go of shame and guilt that may be holding you back from trying new things that you'd like to experience. As a rule of thumb, I suggest trying something new three times. The first and second time, you may be nervous or uncomfortable. If you still don't enjoy something the third time you try it, perhaps it's not for you. That's okay.

COMMON SEXUAL PROBLEMS

I want to talk about some of the most common sexual challenges I see in the men I work with. In later chapters, we'll discuss how to address these issues. For now, I want you to understand that if you're struggling with any of these issues, that's normal. They affect a lot of guys.

The first is **performance anxiety**. Almost every man struggles with some form of performance anxiety at some stage. It comes from our fears about what *might* happen, then we get locked in our minds and can't fully enjoy the experience. We put a *lot* of pressure on ourselves to have epic sex, every time. That's not realistic. Somehow, we absorb the message that sex is a series of moves that we need to get right. When we have a woman in the bedroom, we think we need to throw her around like a porn star, put her in all sorts of different positions, or touch her in a specific way. Although there's some value to techniques, you'll never have great sex if you're stuck in your head.

Meanwhile, the woman you're with is probably putting a lot of pressure on herself, too, locking herself up and reducing the chances of her having an orgasm. You may not know each other well. If you're not communicating, how will she know what you like? How will you know what she likes?

Pressure creates a lot of uneasiness, when sex is really an experience to be shared.

Performance anxiety usually manifests in one of three ways: **erectile dysfunction (ED)**, an inability to get it up or keep it up; **premature ejaculation (PE)**, a tendency to cum too quickly; or **delayed ejaculation (DE)**, difficulty in cumming at all. There's no doubt that poor diet, lack of exercise, and limited sleep all have an influence on these problems. If you're stressed out with work, the kids aren't sleeping, and you're not getting enough downtime, you'll likely find it hard to be interested in sex. Even taking all these factors into account, though, the pressure we put on ourselves has an additional impact. We tend to think that, as men, it's normal to be rock-hard on command. We expect that whenever a woman is ready to go, we should be too.

It doesn't work like that. The more we try to force ourselves to be turned on, the more likely it is that we'll struggle to meet those expectations. Turn-on starts in the mind and spreads to the body; an anxious mind is no recipe for a rock-hard cock. If I came to your house, put a gun to your head, and told you to get it up, would you be able to? I doubt it. But, psychologically, many of us are doing that to ourselves, demanding that we perform under pressure and then feeling guilt and shame when we can't do that. We put ourselves into fight-or-flight mode then beat ourselves up for not performing under pressure.

Think about a time when you've been with a woman you really cared about. Were you worried about getting it up? Probably not. You felt relaxed and in tune with her and found it easy to get turned on. There's a powerful connection between your head, your heart, and your cock. When all three of those forces are aligned, you won't need to worry about performance.

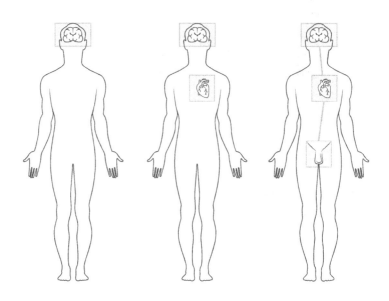

A lot of guys worry about the appearance of their penis. They fear that the size or shape is abnormal. Now, I'm not going to tell you that size doesn't matter at all. If your cock is the size of a grain of rice, you may have some issues. But the range of what constitutes normal is much larger than most men realize. Women who really like you will appreciate your cock as an extension of who you are. If you are on the small side, there's a lot you can do to satisfy a woman.

You can use your hands to touch her. You can use your mouth. You can bring out the sex toys. You can talk dirty and exercise psychological dominance, which we'll discuss further in Chapter Six. You can turn a woman on with role-play and sexual fantasies. When you do all of those things, women will be just as satisfied as they would if your cock were larger, and they'll be having too much fun to focus on size anyway. Whereas if you get hung up on size and shame yourself, you'll give women the impression that you're trying to hide your sexuality, which will likely turn them off.

And by the way, don't worry that a woman's going to leave you for a sex toy. Just see it as an extension of your arm. Pro tip: the best toy on the market is the Magic Wand. For a free training on how to use the Magic Wand, check out sexualquantumleap.com/resources. Pretty soon, you'll be better with a wand than Harry Potter.

Guys will go to any extreme to make their cock bigger. They'll try creams, pills, and jelqing (penis extension exercises). You can do those things. They might even work. But what I want you to understand is that your penis is an extension of your heart. Instead of thinking that you need to have a huge cock for a woman to feel any pleasure, accept what you've been given and work with that. When you connect your heart and your cock, women will feel it. At SQL, we encourage guys to "fuck her in the heart."

Practically speaking, there are positions you can use that will make you feel bigger, but the real antidote to anxieties about size and shape is to appreciate your penis. Scientists have experimented with rice, showing that sending good vibes to rice plants causes them to grow, while sending anger and bitterness to the same plants causes them to shrivel and die.

When you love your cock, women will love it too. I've known guys who were considering corrective surgery because they were worried about the shape of their cock. But there was nothing to "correct." The only thing wrong with them was the belief that something was wrong. Another consideration: the bend of your cock might even enhance a woman's sexual experiences with you. Perhaps it really hits the spot for her. Bottom line: the size and shape of your penis does not determine your worth as a man. Only your character does.

Another major issue a lot of guys encounter is **porn addiction**. Although there's nothing morally wrong with watching porn, it gives a false impression of what sex is like. Some men get lost in a fantasy of how women get turned on and experience sex and get fixated on that fantasy when they're with real women. They start to believe that they need to emulate everything they've seen on porn, or—worse—tell themselves that, because they don't look or fuck like porn actors, they can never truly satisfy a woman. This causes a lot of sexual dysfunction and performance anxiety. There's a reason the people in porn are called actors.

Another problem with porn is that guys get overstimulated. Soon, watching one scene isn't enough. They have ten or fifteen or twenty tabs open. They start looking for more extreme stuff. Soon, they may lose the ability to get turned on by being with one woman. They'd rather jack off to porn than be with a woman. If your brain is wired to expect high levels of stimulation, you'll struggle to enjoy being caressed gently by one woman. You may start viewing women as objects for your sexual pleasure.

There are a couple of exceptions to the rule that watching a lot of porn isn't healthy. It can be a turn-on to watch with a partner. Find out what she likes and watch it together. As she gets turned on, take that momentum into the bedroom. Another way to enjoy it is by filming yourselves having sex and watching it back together. That can be a great way to connect. If you're watching it on your own, try slow porn, which doesn't leap straight to the fucking. It's a way to experience some degree of buildup, as opposed to going straight for the jackhammering or epic blow job scene.

If you only watch porn a few times a month, it's not a big deal. There's certainly nothing morally wrong with it. Unless porn is causing your life to deteriorate or becoming a substitute for a healthy dating life, don't beat yourself up. Personally, however, my life has improved dramatically since I cut it out. If you're worried you might be watching too much porn and you want to destroy your porn addiction, visit sexualquantum-leap.com/resources.

I could write a whole book about performance anxiety, dysfunction, size, and porn. For now, though, the message I want you to take away from this chapter is that you're normal and—most importantly—you're not alone. Whatever you think about your sexuality, you're not crazy. Loads of other guys feel the same way, and they're normal too.

When you realize you're not fucked up, you can start to relax and enjoy sex. A big part of that is simply slowing down and fully experiencing the sensations in your body. When you're with a woman, enjoy teasing her and playing with her. Give her body—and yours—time to warm up. Instead of pressuring yourself to make something happen, concentrate on going as slowly as you can.

Sex isn't supposed to be perfect or look a certain way. It can and should be fun, playful, messy, and explorative. Take the time to build sexual tension, express how you feel, and encourage the woman you're with to express how she feels. Most importantly, get out of your head and into your body.

BRANDON'S STORY: PART II

Brandon's a perfect example of what's possible. He was as good as his word. He gave the retreat everything he had. One of the exercises we do at the retreat is practice fingering a doll. It might sound weird, but if you can put 100 percent of your attention on fingering a doll, imagine how present you'll be when you're fingering a living, breathing woman. Brandon was totally there for it, present, intense, and determined.

On the last night of the retreat, we usually wrap up around 8:00 p.m. This time around, we ended up running late. We were there until 1:00 a.m. Everyone was pretty amped up and we had a model in—we get a model in for retreats so guys can feel how women respond to their presence. We do some crazy exercises that I'm not going to share here! Brandon was shooting the shit with the other guys and admitted that he felt really nervous about kissing.

Normally, the men on retreats don't kiss the models, but I asked Amy—that was her name—whether she was cool with it. "Yeah, fuck it," she said. "I'll do it." We put on different types of music to create a range of different moods and Brandon experimented with kissing her.

At first, he was totally stuck in his head. He kept breaking away and saying, "I feel so stuck. I don't know what to do." Eventually, I told him to shut the fuck up, feel the music, and kiss her like she's the last woman on the planet. So, he did. He walked up to her and started kissing her gently, then pressed her against the wall and made out with her more aggressively. He flowed through softness and assertiveness, while she gave him feedback on her experience.

When they finished, he almost broke down. He had tears in his eyes. He thanked me profusely for setting up the experience, and Amy for sharing it with him. Brandon left the retreat with a totally new understanding of how to connect with women.

Fast-forward a few months and his life had changed dramatically. He went from having zero women in his life to seeing five different women. He felt free to explore what he wanted and express himself authentically. Rather than feeling needy, he enjoyed opening up to women and developing a genu-ine connection—and found that, contrary to his fears, they *wanted* to be around him. Even his relationship with his parents improved, as he found the courage to open up to them more.

In a few short months, his mindset shifted dramatically. Suddenly, he was focused on how he could make an impact in the world, how he could connect with a group of friends who understood and supported him, and the amazing connections he was enjoying with women. Brandon went from being riddled with performance anxiety, convinced that he was fucked up, to knowing and appreciating the shit out of himself. When we spoke, he told me he hardly recognized the scared, frustrated person he'd been prior to the retreat.

2

SIX SEXUAL MINDSETS

Caleb was a real high achiever. He ran his own team of salespeople and was fascinated by personal development. His whole life, he wanted to get better. Despite his success, Caleb was a humble guy, quick to praise others and admit to his failings.

He reached out to me after he saw a post of mine on Facebook and read through the Sexual Quantum Leap website. The first time I spoke to him, it was clear that he was confused. For all his successes, there was a reservoir of dissatisfaction and frustration in his sex life. He didn't know why it wasn't better, or how to improve it. For Caleb, international travel was no big deal. And, at his level of success, the cost of the retreat was well within his budget. His major concern was whether the experience he had on the retreat would be worth his time.

Caleb wanted to improve his sex life, but he didn't want to waste time and money on a substandard experience. After we talked, it didn't take him long to decide to make the leap.

He even brought his partner along. She stayed around the corner, so they could try out everything he learned together as soon as the retreat was over.

His biggest epiphany was that he shut down his own sexuality. He had been doing it for so long that it seemed normal to him. When he and his partner first got together, he was open, explorative, and wild. He loved sharing her desires and listening to what she wanted. They lived out epic sexual fantasies and adventures together. As they got closer, however, he experienced a paradigm shift. No longer was she a woman he was dating. She was his girlfriend. Perhaps, one day, she would be his wife, even the mother of his children.

In Caleb's mind, that set up a conflict. He found it increasingly hard to be uninhibited with a woman he was growing to love. Suddenly, instead of encouraging her to open up sexually, he started shutting her down. Unconsciously, he felt that certain behaviors were only appropriate with a casual partner and became taboo in a serious relationship. The more he fell in love, the more he unconsciously pushed his partner away sexually.

Caleb was on a slippery slope. If he continued on the same path, he was going to create problems in his relationship. Ironically, he was alienating the woman he loved. Outside of a relationship context, he felt free to be wild and fully expressed. Within a loving relationship, he was filled with judgment about his sexuality—and his partner's. Sex was becoming stale and boring, and neither he nor his partner felt truly satisfied.

His partner hadn't changed. She was still as open as she had been when they first got together. In fact, she was willing to explore her wild side with him. But Caleb told himself that it wasn't okay to connect in that way with a woman he loved. No doubt his Catholic upbringing played a part in those beliefs. According to his sexual story, wives and mothers held a sacred position, which wasn't compatible with crazy sexual experiences.

Although he had a really cool exterior, Caleb went all in the moment he walked into the retreat. In his business life, he was a coach and a teacher, but he was willing to let go of that control and be the student. I knew shit was about to get real. And it did.

One of the biggest pieces of work we did at the retreat was rewiring the conflict between his sexuality and his beliefs about relationships. He saw how he was shutting his partner down, how his love for her and his willingness to encourage her sexuality were moving in opposite directions. I made it crystal clear to him that he didn't need to hold on to that conflict. He could love her, support her sexual expression, and simultaneously allow his own sexual expression to shine through.

It was a bitter pill. When Caleb clearly saw how he had been shutting down his girlfriend, he put his hand to his head and screamed, "Fuck!" I asked him about the last time he'd told her he loved her while they were having sex, about the last time he had opened up and told her what he wanted, about the last time he had taken her into the bedroom and really ravished her. "I haven't done that for more than six months," he admitted.

GET INTO YOUR BODY

Fighting, fucking, and dancing. Three things that all men think they're great at...until reality intervenes. The good news is that anyone can get better. Sex starts in the mind, and most men don't have a clue what's possible.

In this chapter, we'll discuss a range of sexual mindsets to get you out of your head and into your body: the first step to deep connection and pleasure. Really great sex is two bodies moving in a rhythmic dance. It's not about one person doing something to another person. It's not about looking a certain way. It's about the energy created by deep connection. It's a flow.

If you've never asked a woman for honest feedback, you may have no idea whether you're good in bed. I didn't, until I got told I was shit in bed, and it woke me up. It was like getting a slap in the face. But it changed the path of my life for the better.

The paradox is that, to get out of your head and into your body, you first need to embrace a shift in mindset. In time, the mindsets we discuss in this chapter will become intuitive and you won't need to think about them consciously, but at first, you'll need to focus your attention on learning them, so that they inform the way you hold yourself, and the way you move. Let's get started.

MINDSET ONE:
SEXUALITY STARTS WITH YOU

You're probably familiar with the idea that personal development always starts with you. It's true of sexuality, too. If you're a good guy, you've maybe got the idea that pleasing women is important. And it is. Better to care about her pleasure than to be a jerk who's only interested in getting his rocks off.

But a lot of guys go too far the other way. We become so focused on her that we forget about our own experience. We lose track of what turns us on and what we want to explore. Your pleasure is important too. The best sex is a shared experience, with both people feeling great. This problem is extremely common among high-achieving businessmen. They lose touch with their own sexuality and don't have a clue how to ask for what they want.

Recently, I spoke to a top-five business consultant in Australia, an exceptional man who specialized in helping businesses scale past a million dollars. He had spent more than a million dollars on his own personal and professional development without ever looking into his sexuality. Over the course of a twenty-minute chat with me, he broke down and cried because he realized that he'd neglected this vital aspect of his life.

It's totally okay to have a night dedicated to pleasuring your woman. That can be fun and sexy for both of you. The problem comes if you lose track of what you like and want. When you understand your own sexuality and you can express it, that demonstrates confidence. Women will see that you're a man who knows what he wants. Your unapologetic attitude to your sexuality will help her feel safe to open up to you. If you can't do that, you'll grow resentful. Much as you enjoy pleasing your woman, you'll gradually become dissatisfied. Women will feel that, too, and instead of opening up, they'll shut down. They won't trust you.

Sure, you want to be the best she ever had. But you also want sex to be the best *you* ever had. If you are constantly trying to give a woman great experiences, she may love you for it, but your inner accountant will be screaming, "What about *my* pleasure?" Don't forget to please yourself. When you are truly doing that, she will see how much you let go and it will turn her the fuck on.

I work with plenty of men who are engineers, accountants, and programmers. They're used to seeing the world in a mathematical way, and they want sex to conform to the same principles. If she does X, I'll do Y. If she says this, I should say that. But sex isn't a formula.

Tattoo this concept on your forehead: every woman is different, every pussy is different. Do it backward, though, so you can read it in the mirror. Some women like things that other women really *don't* like. Sometimes the same woman will love something one day and dislike it another day. Every time you have sex, her mood will be different. She'll be at a different point in her cycle. She may have different desires. She'll feel different after a hard day at work. Hell, she may have eaten something that disagrees with her. It's not possible to plug women into a spreadsheet and get predictable results. We'll talk much more about this in Chapter Five.

If you want to know what works for your woman, ask her! A great way to calibrate is to ask whether she wants you to go higher or lower, faster or slower, softer or harder. Want to do something? Check in with her. Keep checking in, verbally and visually. If you don't ask, you may not know whether she's screaming with pain or pleasure.

One guy, Adrian, came to a Sexual Quantum Leap retreat and got incredibly stuck in his head because he was focused on doing the right things in the right order, rather than thinking about flowing and connection. Part of it came from his upbringing—his dad was constantly telling him he wasn't good enough, and he became a perfectionist. Unfortunately, that strategy doesn't work with women. There's no such thing as the perfect move for the perfect pussy.

He had a very traditional view of masculinity. Don't talk about sex. Play sports. Get a good education—in engineering, in Adrian's case. Adrian put a great deal of pressure on himself. He didn't believe that he deserved to be with a beautiful woman. His dad's message that he wasn't good enough sunk in deep. Not surprisingly, he struggled with getting it up and keeping it up, and became stuck in his head when he was with a woman.

He suffered with analysis paralysis. In Adrian's mind, there was an acceptable way to speak to women and an unacceptable way. If he ever crossed that line, he would recoil like he'd run into an electric fence. On the retreat, when he was doing exercises with a doll, he was stiff and rigid, as though he were trying to figure out the right sequence of moves to unlock a safe.

Sex is a dance of logic and emotion, art and science. He was fixated on the logic. It may seem absurd practicing on a doll, but I always tell guys who come on a retreat that if they can bring their full presence to a doll, they're going to be *amazing* when they have a real woman in their bed. Adrian needed to engage his heart, not only his brain. He was obsessed with trying not to make mistakes, but there'll always be mistakes when it comes to sex. It's messy.

With the assistance of coaching and music, Adrian was able to stay present and flow with the doll. He accepted he wasn't going to get everything perfect, and yet, paradoxically, he enjoyed himself much more. The doll was pretty into it, too. These days, Adrian has no problems getting it up and has met the love of his life.

MINDSET TWO: SEX IS A JOURNEY

A few years ago, I met a brilliant teacher at a sexuality workshop who has been working in sexual education for more than thirty years. I asked her about the end goal of sex. "It never ends," she told me. "It's a constant exploration of what you like and what you want to do." That was a big inflection point for me.

Like a lot of men, I tended to think of sex in terms of reaching a goal—that goal being my orgasm. I took a "get it done, hit and run" approach. We get stuck on that idea and become rigid about what we think we'll like. Of course, this turns women off, too. Before long, sex is the same every time. But it doesn't need to be. It can be a canvas of exploration, without concerns about time and outcome. Think of sex as a place where time and space collapse, and where you can play and have fun. There's no need to force it to be a certain way. It's fluid.

With this mindset, sex becomes an open-ended experience to share with women you care about. The more comfortable you become with each other, the more deeply you connect. You can keep opening up, sharing your desires, peeling off layers. It's an endless process, and it can keep getting better and better.

The same teacher told me that she didn't have any sexual fantasies. I couldn't believe it. "What do you mean, you don't have any fantasies?!" She explained that she had explored them all. She'd given herself so much permission to explore her sexuality that all her fantasies had become realities. If any other fantasies arose, she knew she could give herself permission to explore those, too.

Sex is a never-ending cycle of desire, exploration, and enjoyment. You might not like everything you try, and that's okay too. But don't shut yourself down. Don't shut your partner down. Open your mind to the possibility that there's so much out there for you to explore, more than you could even imagine.

I talk to a lot of men who are looking for cool, sexually liberated women. They don't realize those women are all around them. This book is teaching you how to unlock that side of them in a way that they thank you for. Whatever you're into, I guarantee you there's a woman out there who wants to explore it with you. If you don't fully own and express your sexuality, how will she know?

Once you open up and start to trust your own sexual expression, you'll find that the women you were looking for were right there all along. Sexuality starts with you. When you get clear on what you want, and become comfortable talking about it, you'll attract women who share your interests.

Admittedly, we sometimes get attracted to crazy chicks. I used to see a chick whose special birthday request was for me to fuck her in a graveyard. One time, while we were driving, I made a joke about something. She responded by pulling a knife and holding it five centimeters from my neck while a friend of ours sat in the back seat, goggle-eyed with fear. "Babe," I said, "Two things: one, don't pull a knife on me when I'm driving; two, don't pull a knife on me at all."

"I wouldn't have done it if I didn't love you," she retorted. That night, we had amazing sex.

Most of the time, however, it's better for our health and sanity to steer away from the crazy ones.

The Crazy Ones

In 1997, Apple released their now famous "Think different" ad, with Steve Jobs narrating the following passage that pays tribute to the idea of thinking differently:

> Here's to the crazy ones. The misfits. The rebels. The troublemakers. The round pegs in the square holes. The ones who see things differently. They're not fond of rules. And they have no respect for the status quo. You can quote them, disagree with them, glorify or vilify them. About the only thing you can't do is ignore them. Because they change things. They push the human race forward. While some may see them as the crazy ones, we see genius. Because the people who are crazy enough to think they can change the world, are the ones who do.

I had some fun adapting that speech here as a reminder to stay away from crazy women:

> Here's to the crazy ones. The strippers. The rebels. The coke queens. The round pegs in the square holes. The ones who will pull a knife on you and be emotionally abusive. They're not fond of rules, and they have no respect for you. You can quote them, disagree with

them, glorify or vilify them. About the only thing you can't do is ignore them. Because they change things. They set you back mentally, emotionally, and financially. And while some may see them as the crazy ones, we see them as sexual addictions, wrongly perceived as love. Because the women who are crazy enough to key your car and fuck your brother, are the ones who do!

Next time you feel the urge to get involved with a crazy woman, read this speech and get inspired not to! RIP Steve Jobs, thanks for inspiring me to think differently and change the world with SQL.

Next time you're with a woman, take a second. Breathe her in. Look at the beautiful, unique human being you're sharing a bed with. Enjoy the fact that she's opening up to you sexually. She's showing you a deep part of herself that she may not show many people.

You can find a lot more pleasure from going slowly than you can from rushing through sex to get to the orgasm. The average ejaculatory orgasm lasts between three and six seconds. Whereas sex can last for hours if you want it to. The slower you go, the more pleasure you'll feel. When you *do* finally orgasm, you'll explode like a firework, because you've built up so much sexual tension. The greater the buildup, the bigger the payoff.

A mantra we'll return to frequently in this book is breath, sound, movement, and vocal expression (BSMV). When you're with a woman, breathe deeply and fully to feel more. This will also help her to pick up on your emotional state. Express yourself through sounds, so she can hear how much you appreciate her. Move your body in a way that expresses the full range of your pleasure. To really open up your body. Finally, tell her in words what's turning you on. These four principles are key elements of sexuality. Together, they will allow you to get into your body, become super present, and feel way more pleasure, so that you feel truly alive.

MINDSET THREE: PRESENCE TRUMPS PERFORMANCE

There's no need to get hung up on getting it right. Your full presence is more attractive to a woman than you mechanically going through the motions, trying to get it right. We all want to be truly met by another human being and seen for who we are. Imagine this: when you kiss a woman, you're wholly focused on her. You're not thinking about what comes next or what you need to do tomorrow. You're truly with her.

Has a woman ever asked you "What are you thinking?" when you're in bed together? Or "Where are you?" If that happens, it's a clue that you're not fully focused on being with her. Maybe you're thinking of someone else or tuned out for some other reason. You might even be fucking a woman you're not that into, for the validation or just because it feels better than not getting laid at all. If that happens, she'll feel it. You won't be totally into her, and she'll know.

In the long run, this will cause a massive rift between you. If you don't want to be with her deep down, she will feel your disconnection. She won't trust you. She'll be more reserved and anxious. She'll question you a lot. You will feel shut down and unable to be present.

The same thing can happen to women. Have you ever been in bed with a woman and felt her attention drifting? Perhaps you panicked and blamed yourself. The best way to draw a woman into presence is to be present yourself. Call it out. Have a conversation and ask her what's up.

It could be something simple: maybe she's forgotten to feed the dog or needs to message a friend about plans for the weekend. If there's something urgent, encourage her to take care of it. Otherwise, let her know that there's nothing more important right now. Get her to turn her phone off so she can fully relax. Bring her focus back to the present moment. Most things can be paused for a few hours and revisited later, in service of having a beautiful experience right now. The line, "There's nowhere to be and nothing to do. I got you," has saved my night many times!

What are you like when you're hanging out with your buddies? Chill, funny, confident? What happens when you're in the bedroom with a woman you like? Do you show the best side of yourself, or do you clam up, feeling stiff and awkward? It's weird how quickly we stiffen up—and not in a good way— around women we like. We think we need to act a certain way. Sometimes, the transformation happens between the bar and the bedroom. We're having fun, joking around, and then we get to the bedroom and all of a sudden we're tense. It's a phenomenon I call Robocock.

Jordy is a French rapper who worked for Google. When we met, he was stiff and rigid in bed, and found it difficult to express his natural personality. Following a retreat, he allowed the jokey side of himself to come out more in bed, to the amusement of the woman he was with. "Just shut up!" she said, playfully. They laughed about it and ended up having such great sex that they broke the bed.

If you're a fun guy, don't stop being fun when you get naked. Allow your natural expression to shine through. Say what's on your mind, whether that's words of softness and intimacy or a more animalistic sexual expression. I'm not a fan of the phrase "dirty talk." It implies that sex is dirty. I prefer "sexual expression." Allow it to flow through you. Be loose enough to play.

Tell her you love her, if it's true. Tell her what you find sexy about her. Don't be afraid to look her dead in the eye while you're inside of her and tell her how much you care. Look closely and really *see* her, as a unique expression of a unique person. "You have no idea how sexy I find you." "I love the way you're touching me right now." "I like X about you; it makes me feel Y." "Look how hard you're making me." If you want and you have her consent, take it darker. Maybe, in the bedroom, you like to call her a whore or a slut, and she enjoys it too.

These are just examples. Don't copy the exact phrases above but do be willing to share your experience and make a verbal connection. Do everything in the bedroom with 100 percent presence. Give yourself permission to tap into all aspects of your personality, from your softer side to your primal desire. It'll bring you and the woman you're with closer together.

Exercise:
The Chocolate Test

This is a simple way to bring more presence into your life. Get a bar of chocolate, break off a piece, and eat it. While you chew, think about whatever you feel like. Dinner, what you're going to watch on Netflix tonight, any old random bullshit.

Now, break off another piece, but this time bring your whole presence to tasting the chocolate. Imagine it's the last piece of chocolate you'll ever eat. Swish it around with your tongue so it fills your mouth. Make *love* to that damn chocolate.

What was the difference? Did you really taste the chocolate the first time? Probably not, right? I mean, you enjoyed it, but you were missing so much subtlety that only came through when you gave it all your attention. The same principle applies to being in bed with a woman.

MINDSET FOUR:
SEX IS NOT SIMPLY COCK PLUS PUSSY

A lot of guys think that sex starts when a cock enters a pussy. For a woman, sex starts the moment you catch her eye. You need to warm up her mind before she'll open up her body. Even in the bedroom, it starts with foreplay, building up to deeper levels of arousal.

Talking about sex can be almost as hot as doing it. That's why it's so important to understand your kinks, fantasies, and desires. When you understand what you want to explore, you'll allow the woman you're with to relax too.

It can be incredibly liberating and erotic to tell someone what you want to do with them, or to them. Sex can lose a lot without the sense of anticipation that comes with slow escalation, flirting, and verbal expression. The more you build up a sense of connection and shared understanding, the more sensation you'll feel and the stronger both your orgasm and hers will be.

MINDSET FIVE:
WOMEN LOVE SEX

It's weird how, in the West, we've developed this idea that women are angels who don't like sex, and who recoil when men talk to them in a sexual way. Consent is essential, of course, but the idea that women are sweet and innocent, with no interest in sex, couldn't be further from the truth. If you haven't yet, I recommend that you read Nancy Friday's book *My*

Secret Garden, which is a collection of real sexual fantasies. It will blow your mind. Also, pick up some women's erotica—essentially porn for women.

On "Yeah!," Usher sings about wanting a woman who's a lady in the street and a freak in the bed. He's got it right, yet so many men convince themselves that women are delicate snowflakes with no sexual fantasies or libidos of their own. It couldn't be further from the truth. For the most part, women *love* being sexual. They want to come out and play, and to be seen as sexual beings. But women usually only show this side of themselves to men who are comfortable with their own sexuality, who they can trust not to judge them. The problem is that, if they get shut down, it's more likely that they'll hide their sexuality due to a fear of being judged.

Way too many men out there are slut-shaming women, which sends the message to women that there's something wrong with expressing themselves sexually. It's crazy that we call promiscuous men studs, but denigrate promiscuous women as sluts—a total double standard. For women, being called a slut feels as bad as it does when someone calls you a loser.

As a man, you have a responsibility to encourage the natural, free sexual expression of the woman you're with. Let her know that you won't judge her. When she opens up, accept her and encourage her. Do this consistently, and you'll notice that she relaxes in your presence. She'll be different: more responsive, more expressive. Women are naturally highly sexual, but when they're shut down, they hide their sexuality away.

When you accept a woman sexually, and give her the freedom to be herself, you'll see and hear things you may never have seen and heard before. She'll want to do things in the bedroom that you may always have dreamed of, even if you didn't think they were possible. In her mind, you'll become a beacon of sexual positivity, and she'll naturally gravitate toward you.

Women have many sexual moods. Some days she may need to be touched gently and cuddled. Other days she may need to be pinned down and fucked hard. If you can see her and accept her in all her colors, you'll get an incredible response.

Another thing to consider here is that, sadly, a lot of women have had negative sexual experiences, from rape to abuse. If a woman is initially resistant to opening up, maybe it's because she's still influenced by something from her past. Again, being the guy who can hear that and fully accept her can be exceptionally powerful and healing. Come from a place of genuine care, let her know that you're there for her, and reassure her that there's nothing she can say that will offend you. She just may be ready to open up.

I don't seem like the kind of guy who would go on a cruise, but I have done it. My granny took me on a forty-six-day cruise halfway around the world. On the boat, I was chatting with a woman by the pool and she said, "If you can unlock this"—she pointed to her head—"you can have anything you want from me." A woman's most potent sexual organ isn't her pussy. It's her mind.

For me, the cheeky smile is a secret weapon. It's as though I'm saying to a woman, "I know your secrets," with no more than a look. A lot of sexual communication is nonverbal. You can fuck a woman's soul with eye contact, even while talking about something as mundane as the weather.

Be willing to build sexual tension through holding yourself as a sexual man. Make eye contact and allow her to break it first. Play with her, tease her, gauge her interest. Pull back if you need to. Let her know that you're cool talking about sex without pushing a sexual agenda on her. Move closer to her and feel the tension grow between you. Even doing that will put you ten steps ahead of the average guy.

MINDSET SIX:
WOMEN LOVE A DOMINANT MAN

We'll talk more about dominance in Chapter Three. For now, know that women love a man who can lead, because it allows them to relax. Dominance isn't controlling another person against their will. It's exercising leadership.

At the extreme, consider how many women believe that they're in love with rapists and serial killers. Those guys get an incredible amount of mail from women professing undying love. Exhibit B: how many women have fantasies about werewolves, vampires, pirates, and Christian Grey?

What's the appeal? Why the fuck would women go crazy for rapists and murderers? There's a wildness about them. It's easy for a woman to imagine that a man like that will take them and do exactly as he pleases with them, and that he's willing to do anything to protect her. She, in turn, will have nothing to do but switch off her thinking mind and surrender totally to her sensations. For millions of women, that's an incredibly hot notion. They're drawn strongly into the reality of a man who knows what he wants and goes for it.

Take the example of Jeremy Meeks, who became famous as the world's hottest felon. Women from around the world went crazy for him, despite the fact that he was a former member of the Crips who was convicted of a violent assault on a sixteen-year-old boy.

Obviously, I'm not advocating that you do anything illegal. What I want you to understand is that when you switch on your dominant side, which we'll discuss more later, she will feel like you're taking care of her, she has nothing to worry about, and she can totally relax. This taps into her primal desire to be protected and provided for. Most women melt when a man does this, and they're excited because they've finally found a man who gets it.

The caveat, of course, is that you must use your dominance in service of her best interests. You're not out to aggressively violate her boundaries. Also, realize that dominance doesn't necessarily equate to roughness. You don't need to be six foot three and full of muscles to be dominant. Some of the most dominant men are extremely kind—but not weak. A simple act of dominance could be a look, a request, or a touch. You can be dominant simply by leading her into something she is excited to try but that she may be nervous about.

LEARN MINDSET BEFORE TECHNIQUE

Your sexual mindset is important. If you come into a sexual relationship putting pressure on yourself and trying to force the moment, you're already on the back foot. Slow down, take your time, and enjoy the woman in front of you.

If you get nervous, reassure yourself that women really do love to feel sexual pleasure, especially when they feel totally comfortable with their partner. Women are extremely sexual—not only, as some guys think, when they're drunk or high. A woman who's truly comfortable with her partner will happily enjoy a wild, varied sex life, totally sober.

The mindsets in this chapter are signposts to connection. Apply them as a way to relax. When your internal reality shifts, that'll be reflected in your physiology, which will impact your body language and communication with women. When you show that you genuinely care and invite women to feel safe and comfortable with you, they will gratefully tell you more. They'll want to see you again and share playful, meaningful experiences.

As we discussed earlier in the chapter, however, it's important not to use these mindsets as a crutch. They're a way to become more present, not a manual to refer to. Keep deepening your understanding of your own sexual expression and the sexual expression of the woman you're with. Learn and adapt from moment to moment. Accept that sometimes sex throws up curveballs. Some days you might want it rough.

Other days you could be all about gentleness. In sex, flexibility and discernment will serve you much better than rigidity.

When you approach sex in this way, it will only get better and deeper over time. You will open up to each other more and more, and feel greater intimacy, sensitivity, and pleasure. Sometimes, the best connection comes from not trying. Simply relaxing, lying there with a woman, kissing her and touching her body if you feel moved to, but not making an effort to put on a show or perform. Techniques are useful, and we'll talk about them later in this book, but they're nothing without a mindset that allows you to be present.

CALEB'S STORY: PART II

When Caleb realized he'd been shutting his girlfriend down, he had an epiphany. He couldn't believe that he had an amazing, beautiful, sexually open woman, and he'd been preventing her from fully expressing herself, while simultaneously shutting himself down.

The same night, he called her and said, "Babe, I love you so much. I'm sorry for shutting down the minx inside you who wants to come out and play." It was a huge breakthrough for them both.

Caleb was a changed man when he reunited with his partner after the retreat. They fully reconnected and both of them got to feel heard and seen in their sexuality. She was so amazed that she said she felt as though she was cheating on him with another man. The connection went to a deeper level, as hot as it used to be, but deeper and more connected.

It's hard to sustain great sex in a committed relationship. It takes effort and honesty and communication. Sometimes it's necessary to have uncomfortable conversations. But the payoff is so worth it. Caleb and his girlfriend had started to feel like roommates, as opposed to sexual partners. The spark had disappeared from their sex lives. When Caleb got how he'd been shutting her down, that shifted instantly.

The two of them are still together, although they need to make sure they keep the channels of communication open. Recently, Caleb and I had a chat where he told me that their sex life had taken another minor dip. After we discussed his desires and he went away and talked to her about them, they rediscovered that freshness and excitement.

Caleb, like Adrian, has a tendency to see himself as a provider. When he's stressed, he defaults to feeling as though he's running the show and shuts himself off from requesting support. That can build into resentment. At times, he gives his girlfriend a lot of emotional and financial support, forgets to ask for what he wants, then wonders why he's not getting his sexual needs met. He's found that it's important for him to take time for himself and ask for what he needs.

Sometimes that means having the courage to ask his girlfriend to dress in a sexy outfit, give him a massage, or wake him up with a blow job. His vulnerability opens up the sexual communication between them and heads off the possibility of him becoming too stressed and shutting her down.

Recently, Caleb told me that he and his partner got engaged, and that she's pregnant with a baby girl. Sexual Quantum Leap is having a baby!

3

LEADERSHIP
IS LOVE

When Jamie came to me, he was a typical nice guy. People, including women, tended to take advantage of him, and he was tired of it. Jamie was a self-development junkie, always pushing himself to learn new things and expand his confidence. He also had a bit of a hero complex—subconsciously, he tended to attract women with problems in the belief that he could save them. We've all been there, right?

He met a girl he liked and, at first, the sexual connection was great. Unaware of the red flags she was putting up all over the place, he went all in on the connection. But the more time he spent with her, the more he felt like he was getting lost in her shit. She was mean, even verbally abusive, to the point where he started to lose interest in spending time with her. Some nights, he preferred to stay home playing on his PlayStation. He made up excuses to get out of spending time with her because he knew it would drain him emotionally. But then guilt kicked in. If he left her, who would she have left? That thought always brought him back, and the cycle continued.

He told himself that things would get better. She was going through a rough time. He needed to be understanding. That guy she was messaging all day and night, but who she assured him was "just a friend"? He needed to trust her. The fact that she painted him as a jealous asshole whenever he asked questions about the guy? Maybe he was overreacting. In reality, Jamie was making excuses for her. She wasn't the only person who rode all over him. Jamie found it difficult to assert his boundaries with friends and work colleagues, too. The situation was so bad that Jamie felt himself losing sexual desire for his girlfriend. He became so self-conscious that at times he lost his desire and sex felt like too much effort.

One night, one of Jamie's friends was celebrating a birthday. Jamie's girlfriend had nothing else to do, so—wanting to be a good boyfriend—he ended up inviting her along. Jamie's girlfriend wore sexy, knee-high black heels, and one of the laces came undone as they were walking along the street. "Babe," she said. "Would you tie my lace for me?"

Jamie felt obliged to do as she asked. He got down on one knee in the street and tied his girlfriend's lace. She thanked him by turning to his friends, laughing, and saying, "Yeah, he's my bitch."

The tone of her voice and her body language made it clear that she wasn't joking. She meant what she said. Jamie was stunned. He looked at her as if to say, "What the fuck?" But he didn't say anything out loud. He didn't want to look like a reactive douchebag and bring down the vibe of the evening.

Jamie didn't want to lose his shit and get told that *he* was the one with the problem. He bit his lip and fumed silently.

A month later, the relationship finally fell apart. Jamie was devastated. Worse, his confidence was at an all-time low. His now-ex-girlfriend was an expert at belittling him. He knew she had lied to him frequently, but he thought calling her out would only start a fight and send them into a downward spiral. It was only when they split up that he realized how much her meanness had affected him. Oh yeah, and she started a relationship with the "friend" she was messaging.

With nothing to lose, Jamie reached out to me. We'd met previously during a fourteen-day dating retreat Jamie attended. I gave a seminar that formed part of the course and we made a connection. He loved what I shared and ordered about $300 worth of sex toys from me. Over the course of the retreat, he also connected with a new woman who told him their sexual experience was the best she ever had. Jamie always had potential! We chatted on my Facebook group and occasionally via Instagram. When he hit rock bottom, he figured it was the right time to take the next step. He'd been thinking of coming to a retreat at the end of the year, but suddenly it felt much more urgent. *Carpe diem*, right? Fuck it.

The next retreat was due to take place in Poland, where I was speaking at a dating and personal development summit, prior to running my own retreat. Jamie called me up and asked if we could fit him in. Within twelve hours, he had booked his flights from Australia to Poland. It was a retreat that would radically alter the course of his life.

Even before the retreat started, I sensed that something was wrong. Jamie's a filmmaker, and he had an agreement to do some filming while he was in the country. He showed up in Poland two weeks early, on the understanding that if he did some filming and editing for another guy who was speaking at the summit, he would get free coaching and free entry to the event. Excited by the opportunity, Jamie financed the trip himself, only for the guy to totally ghost him. They ran into each other in a nightclub and the guy didn't even remember who Jamie was. When Jamie asked him about filming, he said, "I already have too many camera-men, but thanks anyway."

Jamie tried to gloss over it, but I could see he was bummed, even if he couldn't admit it to himself. Like a lot of nice guys, he tended to suppress his anger, instead blaming himself and feeling sad. With women, he didn't know how to express anger in a healthy way, so he often took on the burden of their emotions, rather than feel and express his own.

Personally, I'm at the other end of the spectrum. I'm quick to express anger but I sometimes don't realize how sad I'm feeling. On the first day of our retreat, during our sunset break, he told me about his ex-girlfriend and the guy who had let him down in Poland. "I thought I had to shrug it off," he told me. "What would you have done in that situation?"

He might not have been angry, but I was. It pissed me off to see a good dude like Jamie getting shafted. I screamed "fuck!" repeatedly for about ten or fifteen minutes before calming down enough to think rationally. With Jamie's consent, I addressed it with the whole group present, as a lesson in asserting boundaries—and how failing to do that kills sexual attraction.

DON'T FEAR DOMINANCE

We've already touched on the idea that leadership is love. In this chapter, we're going to take it deeper. Dominance equals leadership equals love. I want you to understand how to approach women with a dominant mindset and serve them through your leadership.

First off, let's be clear that everything we discuss in these pages is coming from a place of love. Women love a man who combines vulnerability and empathy with the capacity to step the fuck up and say no when his boundaries are violated. Women will respect you far more when you know yourself and are willing to assert your boundaries. And if you want a woman to deeply fall for you, you need her to respect you. A lot of guys ask me how they can win the respect of women. The answer is that first you need to respect yourself. Respect is fundamental to connection. Without it, you'll find yourself in situations like Jamie's, with women giving you shit, hurting your sexual connection, and messing with your head.

It's great to be a beast in the bedroom, but you have to have a spine too. If a woman feels that she can walk all over you, and that you will agree to her every whim, even when you're putting yourself out and hurting yourself in the process, her pussy will be as dry as the desert.

If women don't respect you, they won't open up to you. You want your woman to greet you at the door wearing a sexy outfit? She'd better respect you; otherwise, forget about it. Women crave a dominant man with high levels of self-respect. Dominant men know what they like and aren't afraid of voicing it, with or without the approval of a woman. Self-assurance is super sexy to women. Also, respect is not a one-time thing. It can increase and dissipate. Women will test you to figure out whether they can trust your self-respect. When they decide you're for real, they'll melt.

In this chapter, we're going to break down the most effective ways to assert boundaries, open up about what you like and don't like, and support a woman in expressing her boundaries. Ideally, you're both coming from a place of understanding, acceptance, and respect.

You'll read about the Three Stages of Sexuality, conflict resolution, and the Care Bear and the Black Bear. When you put these tools into practice, you'll hear women say things like, "Wow, you really get me," "I've never told anyone this before," and, "You know me better than my best friends." Understanding is love in action. A woman can love you but not respect you, or vice versa. Love and respect are the essential combination for becoming a man she can't resist.

Sadly, it's common for guys to think that they can't tell women the truth. What do they do instead? They lie, cheat, or just fail to be truly honest. I did the same, back when I was juggling those three "monogamous" girlfriends, fucking a married woman, and also banging her best friend. I thought I was the man, selling drugs and carrying on behind their backs. Now, I see that behavior as immature and cowardly. I was scared they wouldn't like me for who I was, so I boosted up my ego to make myself feel like the big guy.

Misleading women comes from a scarcity mentality. It comes from fear of losing a woman. Jamie used to try to save the women he was with. But did they really need saving or was that just his perception? (Spoiler alert: It was just his perception.) Meanwhile, who was saving him? Who was standing up for what he needed and wanted?

A word of caution, however. You don't need to be rude or mean when asserting boundaries. Some guys flip from playing the doormat into being an asshole, saying things like, "Fuck you," and "I hate you." They get emotionally disturbed and shout at women. That's not cool or helpful, and it doesn't work. Asserting boundaries is a simple matter of stating what's important to you and expressing what you will and won't stand for. Express your honest truth about important values that you care deeply about. This can be done in a loving way, without aggression.

True leadership comes from being calm, centered, and grounded. It's not excessively emotional. It's the ability to clearly and confidently state where you stand. It's a fine balance. If you're hanging on to a woman who treats you like shit, let her go for the sake of your self-respect. Would you really rather be on your knees, tying a woman's shoelace while she laughs at you than be single and in control of your destiny?

Setting boundaries is simple but not easy. If you feel constricted and shut down in a conversation, check in with that feeling and think about what it has to tell you. It is most likely a sign of your soul getting crushed! In the words of Dr. John Demartini, "I'd rather have the whole world against me than my own soul." Never deny that intuitive voice inside of you.

Hurt people hurt people, and the least you can do as a man is not pass on your pain to others. Know yourself and speak from that knowing. When I need to have a difficult conversation with a woman, I practice what I want to say in the mirror until it feels like second nature. It's not easy to speak honestly and vulnerably, but the rewards are worth it. You can be a nice guy who asserts his boundaries. As a mentor told me, "Don't mistake my kindness for weakness."

THE THREE STAGES OF SEXUALITY

How was your first time? It probably wasn't great, right? Chances are you were nervous as hell, drunk, or high. I'm guessing you were mainly focused on getting your rocks off and being able to tell your guy friends that you'd done it. Were you focused on the woman's pleasure? Or did you put it in for a few minutes, bang away as hard as you could, and wonder why she didn't come back?

There's no shame in doing that kind of thing when you're young and inexperienced. My first time, she sat on top of me, and I lasted less than a minute. I never heard from her again. Ironically, she had the same name as my first sexuality mentor, Shae.

It happens to most of us. But it doesn't feel that great, even for you. It's more of a performance than a shared experience. It's an illustration of the first stage of sexuality, when you're primarily focused on your pleasure. Some guys never grow out of it, and spend their entire lives selfishly chasing their own pleasure, with little thought for the woman. Then, they're surprised when women don't want to have sex with them again.

This used to be me, and it's the reason why I got told I was shit in bed. I know this stage all too well. Stick it in, cum as quickly as possible, then roll over and go to sleep. It's an unconscious approach to sexuality. And hey, it might not even be your fault. Perhaps you learned about sexuality from porn or you're holding on to sexual trauma from the past.

The second stage of sexuality is when guys get focused on the woman. They fixate on giving her pleasure, making her cum, and being "good" in bed. It might seem like an improvement on banging away for your own kicks, but often it's not coming from a very healthy place.

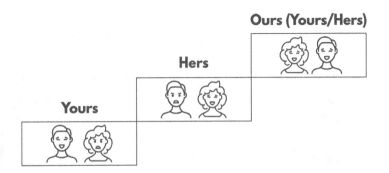

Guys in this stage are sometimes looking for validation. They want to know—and be told—that they did good. Maybe they want the thrill of having a hot girl on their arm. Maybe they want the approval they never got from their mother. There may be an unspoken expectation that the woman will reciprocate. Whatever the deeper reasons, it comes from a lack of self-respect.

It might seem like an improvement to be focused on her pleasure, but it comes with a shadow side. These guys may be bringing out all the party tricks to make women cum, but deep down they're feeling a lot of resentment and dissatisfaction. Sure, she can say it was the best she ever had, but what about you? For every great performance like this, there's a sad little boy inside screaming, "What about me?!"

When you play the game this way, you may be frustrated because your woman treats you like shit, even though you try so hard to please her. Why? Because she can feel that you're not respecting yourself, so why should she respect you? You desperately want her to like you, but you're not willing to express yourself honestly. This dynamic can lead to guys feeling like a performing monkey, constantly trying to give women the best possible sexual experience, while quietly becoming increasingly frustrated.

Like Jamie—and Caleb from the previous chapter—you'll likely build resentment toward her the longer you stay in this stage. Suddenly, you'll decide you're not feeling it for her anymore. You might resort to dysfunctional behaviors, such as going to a hooker, picking up a side chick, drinking, taking drugs, sliding into the DMs of other women, or watching a lot of porn, all in an attempt to cover up your dissatisfaction.

Stage one and stage two are two sides of the same coin. Neither is better than the other. They're both incomplete. Focus on oneself or focus on another person. Some guys start in stage one and move to stage two after they realize they've been selfish. Others do the opposite, trying too hard to please and then thinking, "Fuck it, I'm gonna do what I want."

Stage three is different. In stage three, you're focused on both your pleasure *and* hers. You care how she feels, and you know how to ask for what you want. It's a position of empowerment. When both people in a connection come from this place, sparks fly. Connection becomes a beautiful dance, and the sexual experience is fucking amazing.

You can ask her to do something for you. And you're open to trying things she wants to explore. Your communication is open, honest, and clear. Your connection and level of sexual fulfillment deepen. Instead of stagnating, sex gets juicier and more beautiful.

In stage one and stage two, guys are fairly stuck. They have a limited capacity for relating to women. In stage three, the possibilities are endless. Women know when you're not telling them the truth. If you're consistently untruthful, you're not only lying to her. You're lying to yourself. That will cause you to shut down, limiting your capacity to feel pleasure and enjoy meaningful connections with women.

THE DIFFERENCE BETWEEN DOMINANCE AND BEING DOMINEERING

Simply put, dominance is leading with consent. This is a mutual exchange, with the person being led actively choosing to surrender the power to take charge to someone she trusts. While it may not seem that way at first, the person being led is actually in control. Someone domineering, on the other hand, leads others *without* consent, through manipulation, coercion, and fear, primarily for their own benefit.

Dominance comes from genuinely caring about the interests of someone else. Most women love it when a man takes charge because it allows them to relax, trust that they're in safe hands, and enjoy themselves.

When you grow your capacity for dominance, you'll discover that you can take women to places they've never been before—and they'll willingly follow. It's a common misconception that being dominant requires you to use force. That's not true at all. It's often a lot more understated. She will follow you because she wants to. For examples of dominant men from movies, check out *Secretary* and *The Godfather*.

The key distinction is that dominance is leadership with consent. When you don't have consent, and you try to take a woman places she doesn't want to go, you've stepped into being domineering. Domineering is a form of tyranny. Dominance is benevolent, loving leadership.

Sometimes, dominance is about holding a frame. When you're in the bedroom with a woman, she may get so horny that she demands you fuck her right away. What are you going to do? You don't want to get into a battle of wills, but equally she will lose respect for you if you capitulate. The solution is to hold your frame and reassure her. Grab her tight, put your finger playfully over her lips, make strong eye contact, and say something like, "Chill, I've got you. There's nowhere to be. There's nothing to do."

Additionally, dominance requires knowledge and under-standing. To serve her best interests, you need to *understand* her best interests. To give her great sexual experiences, you need to understand what she likes. There's no point setting up a surprise dinner date at a Thai restaurant if the woman doesn't like Thai food. By the same token, your woman won't thank you for tying her up and spanking her if that's not something she enjoys. The domineering man doesn't care about any of that. He's only focused on getting and doing what he wants, regardless of a woman's interests.

These concepts apply to other areas of life. Do you walk your talk? Do you connect easily with other people? Do colleagues naturally respect you? When you need to set a boundary, do you do it calmly yet firmly? "I don't appreciate that" and "That's not cool" are two lines that have saved me an enormous amount of time. A dominant man calmly lets a woman know when she's crossed a line. A domineering man manipulates and threatens to get what he wants.

CONFLICT RESOLUTION

What happens when a woman disrespects you? How do you respond?

Imagine you're in bed with a woman and she pulls your hair. You're not into it, so you calmly say, "Hey, babe, please don't pull my hair." Now imagine it happens again. You can give her the benefit of the doubt, but make sure she knows it's not cool. "Babe, I just told you I don't appreciate that. Please don't do it again."

If she pulls your hair a third time? That's taking the piss. At that point, you stop, look her directly in the eye, and say, "Why did you pull my hair again?" At this point, she's doing it deliberately, and you need to assert a strong boundary. You still don't get angry, but you want to find out why she keeps disrespecting you. At this point, you expect an apology and a commitment not to do it again.

Then, shut up and wait for her to respond. This is about your self-respect. Whatever happens, you'll win here. You'll retain your self-respect and learn a lot about the character of the woman in front of you. Do you feel a genuine apology? Maybe she got carried away and wasn't paying attention to what you said. It's possible. If so, that's cool, as long as she doesn't do it again. You'll feel the energy shoot up again, and likely the connection will go to the next level.

But what if she's yanking your chain? Is her apology sarcastic or insincere, or does she not bother to apologize at all?

SQL Conflict Resolution Graph

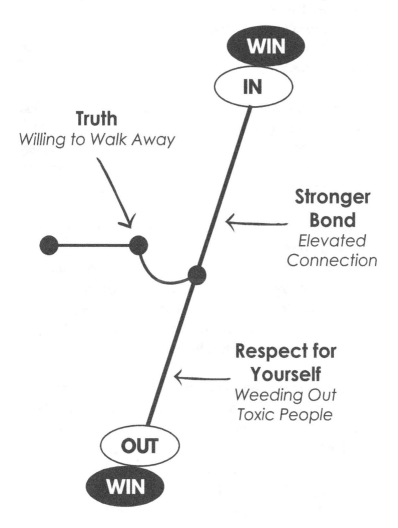

Maybe she tries to make out that it's not a big deal or gives you shit. In that case, maybe you need to leave, or ask her to leave. You don't want to scream and shout or lose your shit (even if she is), but you need to make it clear that you don't tolerate disrespect. Think of the situation as a negotiation, not an argument.

The advantage of this approach is that you get a resolution. You learn something about who she is. If she's got a good character, she'll apologize and you can connect more deeply. If not, you find out early before she can cause you more problems. Believe me, you don't want women like that in your life.

I've had men tell me that this has happened with a woman they love. They're super invested, and they can't imagine setting a boundary like this. I get it. It's difficult to do. The alternative, however, is inviting disrespect into your life. This isn't a relationship book, but if a woman deliberately does things you've asked her not to, there are issues. Unless you resolve them, you'll continue to struggle.

The same principle works the other way. If she says that she wants to stop or slow down, you respect her request. When a woman trusts you to lead her with care, she'll be open to almost anything you suggest. It also applies outside the bedroom, with both male and female friends. Most guys hold on to their frustration when someone violates a boundary. That's a recipe for bigger issues down the line.

A guy I worked with, Greg, experienced this firsthand. A woman he had been seeing for about a month left him hanging for days, even weeks, when he called her. She ignored his calls and didn't call him back, then called after an unreasonably long time, offering an insincere apology but no meaningful explanation. It wasn't until he stood up for himself that he started to see different results. He told her it wasn't cool to ignore him, and she changed her tune. She apologized sincerely and offered to meet up with him. Although the relationship ultimately didn't go anywhere, it was an important lesson for him about respect. Greg is now with a woman who he cares about and respects him.

The issue is that holding on to resentment will kill your satisfaction and pleasure in the bedroom. Have you ever tried to have sex with someone you actively resent? It's not a good experience. Guys come to me all the time complaining that they're not feeling as much pleasure as they want, and it turns out that they're still pissed off about something their partner said two weeks prior. This can continue for months, even years, leading to a buildup of dissatisfaction.

Conflict resolution is a constant practice. It requires repeated back-and-forth. The buildup and release of tension. It also has a direct sexual component. If you don't resolve conflicts in your life, you may become stuck in your head and find it difficult to relax. That stress, in turn, can cause PE or ED, along with more general sexual dissatisfaction, both for you and your sexual partner.

When you call a woman out for disrespecting you, there are many ways she can respond. The six most common are below, in the order they most frequently occur. Your aim is to get to Step 6. You don't want to end a conversation with a disingenuous apology and a feeling, deep down, that nothing got resolved.

A healthy woman shouldn't require you to pass through all these stages. Conflict resolution should be a simple conversation. You may feel a bit distant for a while, then you'll resolve the dispute and feel close, connected, and horny again. On the other hand, some women may cycle through all of these, so it's good to be prepared.

- **Step 1:** Aggressiveness/personal shots (you'll feel distant and not want to touch each other).

- **Step 2:** Playing the victim, perhaps with passive-aggression and fake tears, or by ignoring you.

- **Step 3:** More personal shots; she may run out or try to hit you.

- **Step 4:** Sarcastically saying she's sorry, without really meaning it.

- **Step 5:** Genuine submission and apology (at this point you should feel an ease in your heart and a desire to be close to her again).

- **Step 6:** Arousal and a desire to have sex.

If you don't know how to resolve conflict, it might contribute to damaging your libido, a more common problem than most men think. For a training on getting your libido back, check out sexualquantumleap.com/resources.

THE CARE BEAR AND THE BLACK BEAR

The Care Bear and the Black Bear are two sides of your personality. The Care Bear represents your softness, vulnerability, and caring nature. For example, how do you treat children and animals? Are you kind to them? When your Care Bear energy is strong, women will see you as a reliable man with the potential to be a good father.

Now, let's say you're at the shopping center with your wife and daughter, and a robber runs out of a shop directly toward you. What do you do? Your woman wants to know that, when the shit hits the fan, you can fuck that robber up and bring out your inner warrior to protect your family. It's the Black Bear energy, with no fucking around.

Women need you to bring both the Care Bear and the Black Bear. If you can only bring the Care Bear, she'll see you as nice but unthreatening. She'll likely put you in the dreaded friend zone. By the same token, if you've only got the Black Bear available, she may be attracted to you, but she'll also be scared of you. You won't feel safe to her, and she'll resist letting you lead her to new places.

You're a saint and a sinner, an angel and a devil, Care Bear and Black Bear. If you try to repress one of these aspects, it will come out in other ways. Spend too much time in the Black Bear and you may get burned out. Emotionally, you'll start to harden and lose the capacity for tenderness. Identify too heavily with the Care Bear and you'll feel easily moveable, like a leaf in the wind.

Another way to look at this is through the lens of the masculine and feminine. The Black Bear is the masculine and the Care Bear is the feminine. A woman wants to know that you embrace both the masculine and feminine sides of your character, with the ability to get things done *and* to give and receive care. The ideal is to find a balance, so you can bring both those styles at the right times, inside and outside the bedroom.

GENTLE, ANIMALISTIC, PLAYFUL

I often use this acronym (GAP) as a way to talk about different sexual moods. We've got all three of these experiences inside us, and we bring them out at different times, depending on the environment and the connection.

Gentleness is that sweet, soft, romantic side of you. The side that wants to set up candles in the bedroom, put on chill music, and give her a long, slow massage. Gentle sex can feel amazing, really deep and connected. When you're in a gentle frame of mind, there's nothing to do and nowhere to go. You'll want to take your time, allowing the sexual tension to build until it overflows.

The animalistic mood is much more primal. When you're animalistic, you're tapped into your sexual hunger. Your

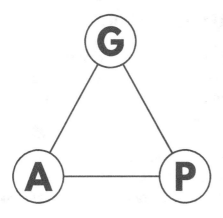

desire's so strong that you want to rip her clothes off and fuck her right there. It's exciting, urgent, and potent.

Sometimes you may need to go animalistic. She may need it too. We all have that side, and we need to let it out. Pin her down or tie her up. Ravish her body. Let her know how goddam much you want her. Whatever crazy noises want to come out of you, let them come. You might want to roar or growl.

Weird as it sounds, a lot of guys are frightened of being playful in the bedroom. You like having fun outside the bedroom, right, so have fun inside the bedroom, too. It's cool to laugh and joke and mess around when that's the vibe between you.

Too many guys have fun outside the bedroom then act as though, when they get behind closed doors, it's all business. Don't shut down your playfulness or take sex too seriously just because you're naked. Embrace it, let it out.

A NICE GUY WITH BOUNDARIES

Summing up everything we've covered in this chapter, it's totally possible to be a good man and simultaneously hold your boundaries. You can be kind, caring, and friendly without being a pushover.

Women need to know that you have a backbone. They want to know that you can ask for what you want and hold your boundaries. In sex, that translates into great communication. Telling her what you like, asking for what you want, and leading her with her best interests at heart.

Sex takes us to our edges. To maximize pleasure, we need the capacity to navigate those edges. When you can ride the waves of sexual pleasure with a woman, giving and receiving feedback, you'll be that nice guy with boundaries.

I like to talk about the idea of the best friend who you fuck. How do you treat your best friend? You care. You respect them. Add in sexual tension, and it's a potent mix. Without genuine care, will you still be friends? Without sexual tension, will you still want to fuck?

My mindset is to build up the woman I'm with as much as possible. I want to make her life better and leave her happier than when we met. Women can feel that intention. Try it next time you meet a woman you like. Ask yourself how you can collaborate with her. There's no need to fight. When you forge a connection, you're in it together.

If you want to lead a woman, you need to claim your own crown. As Conor McGregor put it, "We're not here to take part, we're here to take over." You need to make a stand for who you are and what you believe in. No one will hand you authority. A lot of people are looking for someone to crown them, but the only way to truly feel your own authority is to claim it for yourself.

The question is, how will you lead? Will you lead from love and genuine care? Will you build up the women you're with and make their lives better? Will you build a flourishing kingdom together? Or will you sink into tyranny?

For your sake, and the sake of all the women you meet, I hope you'll choose to be a benevolent leader. There will always be people to support you and people to challenge you. Embrace both and grow into your dominance. True leadership comes from a place of love and service. Leadership is scary as fuck. Sharing your heart and soul with another person is highly vulnerable. But waiting for the other person to go first rarely works. She's likely as nervous as you are. When you open up, you give her permission to do the same.

Be courageous, lean into your leadership. Be willing to open up first and follow the path of most resistance. Only ask people to do things you have done yourself. Understand that when everyone around you is running scared, it's your time to charge forward, with double the force. Live with the heart of a lion, strong enough for a woman to hold on to your mane and ride off into the sunset. For even more on dominance, head over to sexualquantumleap.com/resources and try out the dominance exercise you'll find there.

JAMIE'S STORY: PART II

When Jamie told me how his girlfriend disrespected him, I was livid. I sat him down for a man-to-man chat. I explained that, in Jamie's situation, I would have pulled her away from his friends to prevent a scene from breaking out and let her know that the way she spoke to me wasn't cool. Calmly, with strong eye contact, I'd have told her it's not okay to refer to me as her bitch.

As with the hair pulling example, I'd have been looking for a genuine apology and an understanding on her part that her behavior wasn't acceptable. When Jamie wasn't able to do that, his relationship gradually disintegrated. "Ah fuck," he said. "That's what I should have done."

When the time came for Jamie to finger the doll, he was stuck in his head. He requested the Ed Sheeran song "Shape of You" and approached the doll tentatively. He didn't take charge. I could see exactly why chicks walked all over him. Yeah, the way a guy fingers a doll says a lot about how he shows up in his life. I stopped him and gave him a pep talk. "That's not gonna make a chick's pussy wet, man. How can you get more focused and present?"

He started to get into a flow. The Black Bear came out and he *owned* that doll. It was a real transformation. Reflecting later, he deeply understood what it meant to stand up for himself.

He realized that he'd been walked over by women—and by the guy he came to Poland to meet—because, on some level, he invited it. He was too much of a yes-man.

Ultimately, women will treat you the way you allow them to treat you. That insight shifted Jamie's mindset. He started standing up for what he believes in. He set better boundaries with his work and friends, even his family. He claimed his own crown and put a stake in the ground. No more allowing bullshit into his life. I needed a videographer, so we agreed to work together. We still do. He's become a backbone of Sexual Quantum Leap and my right-hand man.

His connections with women shifted completely. He met an amazing chick who adored him. Later, she admitted—knowing he and I were close—that she didn't want to tell him he was the best she ever had. It felt too cliché. But it was true. I helped him run a small sex party in Brisbane, with about twelve girls and five dudes.

The contrast was like night and day. His new woman never gave him shit for no reason. Their connection was deep, wild, and respectful. Even better, he built a rock-solid confidence, knowing that he didn't need to chase after women. They naturally felt his heart and his strength.

Today, Jamie is one of our head coaches at Sexual Quantum Leap. He knows that whenever he meets a new woman, he'll blow her mind. He's confident opening up, expressing himself sexually, and leading her into new, amazing experiences. Women respect him. He respects himself.

4

KNOW WHAT YOU WANT, ASK FOR WHAT YOU WANT

Colin was in the financial game, with his own business as a mortgage broker. The first time we spoke, he gave off the vibe of being a bad motherfucker. I've worked with a lot of badasses and they fight the hardest against opening up to vulnerability. I knew Colin was going to be a tough nut to crack.

He reached out to me shortly after a divorce. His marriage had ended badly, and he was going through some psychological pain. He was brought up in a Christian cult where his sexuality was somewhat suppressed, and—although he had five kids—his sexual connection with his wife lacked passion. He didn't feel understood, and he'd shut down in response. He was driven and heavily into personal development, and he thought that what I teach could give him an edge in life.

Although he wanted to work with me, I could tell that he was holding back. There was a little boy inside still replaying the tape of the ridicule he received from his mother and sisters while he was growing up, who didn't even know how badly he needed love. He thought that if he trusted a woman, she would manipulate and take advantage of him. He knew how to connect with women sexually, but he was extremely wary of opening up emotionally. Colin wasn't even aware of how much he craved deep emotional and sexual intimacy.

Driven by his unspoken needs and fears, Colin had a high need to be in control. In his mind, the idea of telling a woman that he loved her was crazy. It would demonstrate weakness. His brain was stuck on red alert and he couldn't relax around women. Instead, he played games, both with himself and with women. He was constantly planning his interactions so that he could stay on top, stay in control, and avoid getting hurt. For Colin, connecting with women was about being one step ahead. He saw women more as games than as human beings. His mentality was more suitable for a game of chess than an intimate connection.

It's a common attitude. Loads of men worry that if they open up, they'll get a punch in the gut for their trouble. The idea that boys don't cry and men aren't emotionally available hurts everyone, both male and female.

Colin didn't come to a retreat to crack open emotionally. He wanted to learn techniques that would make him a better lover, so he could gain an advantage over other men. He knew that his sexual experiences weren't as satisfying as he wanted and he felt that, through working with me, he could become the man, sexually. The bigger they are, though, the harder they fall. When he finally let go and expressed his emotions, they poured out of him like Coke fizzing out of a shaken-up bottle.

He admitted that he felt like everyone else was enjoying connection and love, while he was holding women at arm's length because he was terrified of reliving the pain of his previous relationship. Showing his whole heart, including his feelings of unworthiness, felt incredibly scary. He was scared anyone he allowed close to him would take advantage of him.

Sometimes guys without much sexual experience idealize the woman they're with, even if she's an objectively horrible person. Colin went to the other extreme. He learned some pickup game and knew how to attract women, but no one was ever good enough for him. All he could see were their flaws and limitations. He projected his own sense of never being good enough onto the women he met and rejected them before they could reject him.

At the time Colin came to one of my retreats, he was with a woman he'd been seeing for about five or six months. He stubbornly resisted the idea of telling her he loved her, even though he did. "No, man, that shows weakness. If I tell her I love her, she'll have the upper hand." He watched YouTube videos of supposed dating coaches claiming that guys who tell a woman they love her first lose all their power. He used to play songs with the words "I love you" in them, in the hope that they'd trigger her subconscious and she'd say the words first.

Despite these barriers, however, he made it to the retreat. He was a curious combination of humility and arrogance: talkative and opinionated, yet aware enough to realize that he had a lot to learn. I spoke to him before we started, making it clear that I needed him to take off his teacher hat and show up as a student for the duration of the retreat. He's fifteen years older than me, so it may have been hard for him to do, but he did it. He put himself in a receptive state.

The guy knew there were things he didn't know, but he didn't know what they were. He was committed to being better. Lots of the men I work with think they'll only get techniques when they come on a retreat. That's part of it, but there's a deeper component to the work as well. It's both an art and a science. Every retreat is drenched in blood, sweat, and tears; either the clients are crying, or I am—sometimes both. We don't fuck around.

YOUR DESIRES ARE OKAY

Between two consenting adults, no sexual desire is wrong. Maybe you've been told that you shouldn't express or explore the things that truly turn you on. If so, you're not alone. We're all influenced by friends, societal expectations, and the things we see in porn.

But that doesn't mean those influences are correct. No one gets to tell you what you should or shouldn't like. I want to be *super* clear here: as long as you and your partner(s) are all adults and you all give your explicit, unimpaired consent, *no one* gets to tell you how to express your sexuality. Play, explore, and discover what you like.

I work with a lot of guys who are shut down. They're holding on to beliefs about what they're allowed to do and what they're supposed to like, and they hardly dare admit—even to themselves—what they'd like to try. The fundamental issue is not that their desires are wrong. It's that they're too scared to communicate with their partners. Suppressing their true desires causes a lot of dissonance and dysfunction. Fear of being weird ruins a lot more relationships than *actually* being weird.

Here's an example. A prostate massage can feel fucking amazing. But a lot of men shy away from it because they think they'll be considered gay if they admit that they want their partner to touch their prostate. As I mentioned, I used to think this way myself, thanks to a narrow-minded family friend growing up.

Similarly, how many men truly set aside time to masturbate in a way that honors their desires? When a woman plays sensual music, takes a bath, and sets up candles in the bathroom, we tend to think that's fucking sexy. But if a man does something similar, we judge him. You don't *have* to copy that idea—maybe it doesn't do anything for you—but you *could*. You get to pleasure yourself in whatever way works for you. The more honestly you express yourself sexually, the more pleasure you will feel.

If you can't enjoy pleasuring yourself solo, how can you fully experience pleasure with other people? If you don't know your own body, how can you hope to get what you want when you're with a partner? This principle is well known in personal development. It always starts with you; why would sexuality be any different?

Remember, too, that your desires may shift. There may be times when you want a soft, sensual experience, and others when you want to go at it hard. Your desires oscillate constantly, and it's totally okay for them to change day-to-day. The key is to communicate with your sexual partner(s) about what you want to explore and how you want to explore it.

Don't just finish work and jump straight into sex. If you do that, you'll bring your work into the bedroom, which won't be sexy. You probably won't be particularly present and your pleasure will decrease significantly. You don't want to be thinking about spreadsheets and profit-and-loss accounts while making love to your partner. Before having sex, you can look deeply into each other's eyes, breathe deeply together, and verbally set an intention for your lovemaking. At the very least, take a moment to check in before doing the do.

This chapter is all about accessing and acting on your desires, in a way that feels truthful, aligned, and exciting. Don't assume that just because you gave a woman multiple orgasms or made her squirt, she had a great time. Usually it does, but there's so much more to it. You can have sexual chemistry without intimacy, or vice versa. The mix gets truly potent when you have both. Get truly curious about your desires and hers and be willing for sex to look and feel completely different to your expectations.

Realistically, you'll have great sex and shit sex. There'll be days when you're not at your best. If you constantly put pressure on yourself to deliver world-class experiences every time you're together, you'll go into the bedroom tense and anxious. You'll also lose track of your own sensations, which will shut down your ability to be present and feel pleasure. It's a vicious circle.

You might think that clear communication isn't sexy. But the truth is that it will allow the woman you're with to feel safe, trusting, and open. That opens the way for her to feel much more turned on. When you give yourself full permission to talk about your desires, you give her permission to do the same. She may tell you things you never would have believed possible.

Maybe your partner's pretty conservative, and you're assuming that she's not hiding any wild secrets. You may be way off base. I guarantee you that if you unlock that side of her nature, you will see a different side of her personality, one that you never even knew existed. When you do this well, the depth of your sexual connection will only increase over time, and the sex will get better and better.

Of course, it's a risk. She may feel shy and find it difficult to open up. If so, it's your job to be patient. Take the pressure off, be open and encourage her to be open, look at her with love and kindness, and above all don't judge her for what she likes. Over time, you'll see her walls begin to come down.

Choosing Safe Words

I can't emphasize enough that everything I'm talking about depends on informed consent. That means adults who want to be in a sexual situation. Great sex is about two— or more—people allowing themselves to be heard, seen, and understood. It's not about taking what you can get and ignoring the needs of others.

To navigate consent in sexual situations, it's a great idea to have safe words. The most commonly used safe words are "green," "yellow," and "red." Green means carry on doing what you're doing. Yellow means slow down, your partner is getting close to an edge. Red means please stop. Or pick a word you wouldn't normally use in the bedroom, like "avocado."

Taking it one step further, if she's wearing a ball gag or has her panties stuffed in her mouth, she won't be able to clearly say a safe word. In that case, agree on a set of signals, like nodding or shaking her head in a certain way to indicate that she wants to stop. Or moving her hands in a certain way that indicates stop.

It should go without saying that you should always respect and appreciate a safe word or signal. Never get angry, even if you really wanted to keep going. When she calls out a safe word, make her feel fully heard. Acknowledge her for honoring her boundaries. It's essential to validate her expression of her boundaries—otherwise you're teaching her that she can't trust you.

THE PARADOX OF PLEASING

Judging by the movies and magazines, you'd think that all sex is amazing. In reality, it won't be great all the time. Sometimes you'll have incredible sex. Sometimes it won't be that great. Accept that and take the pressure off. You don't have to give a woman multiple screaming orgasms every time you see her.

As we discussed in the previous chapter, your pleasure is as important as hers. If you ignore what you want for the sake of pleasing her, you'll gradually build up resentment. "What about me?" you'll think. Ironically, you'll find her less and less sexy, because you'll be so focused on what you're not getting from the connection.

JAN'S RUBIK'S CUBE FANTASY

I've heard guys talk about almost any fantasy you can imagine. Many of us think that if we tell the truth about what we're into, women will run away, reject us, or think we're the devil. At the same time, we tend to have a skewed perception of what constitutes kink. We hear Rihanna singing, "Chains and whips excite me," and think that defines kink. In fact, kink is whatever you want it to be. Whatever turns you on.

Jan was on a retreat when he told me how much he loved doing a Rubik's Cube. He was crazy good at it; his fastest time was around five seconds. He told me that one of his greatest fantasies was to fuck a girl doggy style while doing a Rubik's Cube, although he didn't think he'd ever get to fulfill that fantasy.

He thought his desire was weird and couldn't imagine a girl wanting to do it. I told him, "No, it's cool, man." He didn't want to hurt anyone. He just wanted to do a Rubik's Cube while having sex. Unusual, sure. But there was nothing wrong with it. I let him know that if he approached a woman with the idea that what he wanted was weird, she'd probably agree. But if he held the frame that it was cool, he'd likely find a chick who was totally into it.

It's not like he wanted to dress her up in a pig outfit with a curly pink butt plug, wearing a Santa hat, and throw tomatoes at her with his right hand while jerking off with his left. And hey, if that's what turns you on, I'm not shaming you; just saying that fucking a chick while doing a Rubik's Cube is a lot easier!

So many guys think that whatever they're personally into is weird. They fear that if they express what really turns them on, they'll be met with shock or humiliation. So, they push their desires down and refuse to admit what they're really into. They feel ashamed of what they like. If it's not straight-up missionary sex, they judge themselves. And, in the process, they rob themselves and the women they're with of amazing experiences.

Alternatively, like Caleb, they compartmentalize their sexuality, only doing certain things with certain women. There's no need for this—the more I love a woman, the crazier the sex becomes!

The day after Jan told me about his Rubik's Cube fantasy, I had him bring out his Rubik's Cube and put on some music. We both kept our clothes on, but I went down on all fours, doggy style, and started yelling, "Oh Jan, come here. I need you to fuck me. I need you to fuck me with your Rubik's Cube in front of the whole class!"

Of course, he burst out laughing. He came up behind me and pretended to fuck me, while everyone else at the retreat cracked up. When he got close to finishing the Rubik's Cube, I started yelling, "I'm about to cum!" as he spanked me on the ass. Suddenly, having sex with a woman while holding his Rubik's Cube didn't seem that weird.

A month or so later, Jan called me to let me know that he'd lived out his fantasy. He sent me a photo—with her consent—of himself and a girl he'd just had sex with. He was holding his Rubik's Cube. Yeah, he did it, he lived out his fantasy. And she loved it! The point here is that even if you think some aspect of your sexuality is weird, there are other people who will be into it. When you find the courage to open up about it, women who care about you will likely respect you—and may want to explore it with you. Think about it: if a woman you were into wanted to try something new with you, you'd be open to it, right? Why wouldn't they feel the same way about you?

RESPECT YOUR BOUNDARIES BUT DON'T BE A DICK

The other side of the coin is that the more you show up for women with no judgment, fully accepting who they are and never pressuring them to do things they don't want to do, the more they'll start opening up to you about *their* fantasies. Sometimes you may be super into their fantasies. Other times, they may not sound good to you.

As guys, we're under a lot of pressure to be sexually adventurous. The more women we sleep with, the cooler we are. The wilder the shit we do, the more other guys look up to us. That's cool, but stay true to yourself. If a woman suggests something you're not into, it's okay to say no.

It's super important, however, to stay respectful. How would you feel if you opened up about a fantasy and a woman replied, "Ew, that's gross!" Don't judge or shame someone for having the courage to share her fantasies with you. If you're not into it, say something like, "Thanks for sharing. I really appreciate you opening up to me. I'm not really down for that at the moment, but maybe in the future that will change."

You can follow up by asking her how she got into this fantasy scenario. Show genuine curiosity and let your facial expressions reflect your interest. You can even ask whether there's anything else that would give her similar satisfaction. Maybe there'll be something you are comfortable with. However you choose to frame it, be as kind and gentle as you can. Let her know that you welcome and appreciate her sexual openness.

THE WAY YOU MASTURBATE IS THE WAY YOU FUCK

Most guys train themselves to be sprinters in the bedroom, like Usain Bolt running a hundred meters in 9.58 seconds. Then, they expect to get with a chick and magically become a marathon runner. It's not going to happen.

Does this sound like you? You started masturbating around the age of twelve or thirteen. Typically, you hid away and were nervous about getting caught. Mom's getting dinner ready and you're on the computer, scrolling through porn and jerking it as hard as you can. Hunched over the computer, body closed off, trying to pop before Mom calls you for dinner.

It's a really tense situation. What you're doing is shutting off a lot of pleasure pathways through the body, training yourself to tense up and cum as quickly as possible. Your ears are on high alert for any noise that could indicate you might get caught. Maybe you're judging yourself for watching porn, thinking that it's bad or wrong, or worried that touching yourself is unnatural (ever heard it'll make you go blind?).

Knowing that your mom could walk in at any moment, you've got your cock in a death grip, going as quickly as you can.

You're more focused on going as quickly as you can than creating a pleasurable experience. You're probably holding your breath or breathing shallowly, as you try to concentrate and hope your mom doesn't call you for dinner—is there anything worse than hearing your mom's voice while you're jerking off? Maybe in Freudian psychology there's a reason why you're jerking off when your mom's around, but let's not go there.

Locked in position at the hips, your body is closed off, super tense and constricted, as is your vocal expression. No breath, sound, movement, or vocal expression here. Plus, no one's ever taught you how to masturbate, so you just bash away. When you do bust a nut, you feel a bit dirty and ashamed.

This might sound like a funny story, but it's also really sad, because when you masturbate, you're training your body's sexual response. You're training yourself to beat off like a beta. Tense, anxious, ready to cum as quickly as possible. Suppressing all vocal expression because you don't want anyone else to hear you. It's not going to translate into a great experience when you're with a woman.

Most of us never break these patterns. As grown men, we still masturbate as quickly and quietly as we can, because we don't want our roommates or kids to hear. We approach masturbation as a quick way to relieve stress, not as a source of pleasure on its own.

What if you made self-pleasure a priority? Set aside time to enjoy it. Allow your breath to flow freely, and make whatever sounds come out of you. Wear something you feel good in. Open up your chest and find a relaxed position, so you can really make love to your body. Scratch yourself with your nails. Cover yourself in coconut oil. Whatever turns you on, use masturbation as an opportunity to take your time and explore what you like. Train your body to welcome and appreciate pleasure. Open up your chest and sit or lie in a relaxed position, so you can make love to your body. You can even take a bath and light some relaxing candles. Don't worry; you won't become gay! For more ideas, check out the guided self-pleasure audio at sexualquantumleap.com/resources.

UNLEASH THE BEAST

Don't suppress your sexual energy. Give yourself permission to explore every aspect of it, from the gentle to the wild, animalistic primal beast. A lot of guys nowadays are divorced from their primal desires, which makes it tough to fully get out of our heads and into our bodies. Sex doesn't have to be pretty; underneath the social conditioning, we're animals. It's okay to express that.

One of my favorite ways to get into a primal headspace is to set up a wrestling date. Find a suitable space in your home, say the living room, and bring out a load of pillows and other soft furnishings. Cushions, beanbags, the bedspread from your bed—whatever it takes to make the floor safe to land on.

Now face your woman, agree that the bout is starting, and launch into each other. Seriously, this is so much fun. Remember when you were a little kid, leaping into ball pits and bouncing on bouncy castles. This is the adult version. Obviously, check in before you start. Agree on safe words. Make sure there are no sharp objects around. But most women *love* this. Many grew up wrestling with older brothers. They'll give as good as they get.

At first, you might be worried about hurting her. As long as you're not being reckless, however, you'll likely discover that she's stronger than you thought. The awesome thing about this game is that it gives both of you permission to tap into your primal, aggressive selves. You might be surprised how much of a badass she is. You may really get into the mood, pretending to be wild animals and making primal noises. Get sweaty, raw, and primal, and give your crazy side permission to come out and play. It's so cathartic to let loose like this.

Of course, there's a high likelihood this will turn into sex. Hold her down for a minute or two and watch how she goes from fighting you really hard to being super turned on, as she feels your strength. You can even start naked, or in your underwear, for extra sexiness. Wrestling is some of the best foreplay I've had. It's an amazing way to test the boundaries and find out exactly how far you can go.

You can start slow and build up gradually, until you're both giving it your all. Bonus: it's great exercise!

COLIN'S STORY: PART II

Colin's ideas of what it means to be a man got turned upside down on the retreat. He thought telling a woman he loved her was weak, but he was forced to admit that the reverse was true. He was weak because he was too scared to admit how much he cared about the woman he was seeing.

During a break, I pulled Colin aside and asked his permission to get 100 percent real with him. When he gave it, I unloaded. "You're a fucking pussy, man. You're so full of shit. You're manipulating women to get a result, but inside you're fucking scared. Have some balls and tell this woman how much you love her."

That might sound extreme, but I could tell Colin needed a shock to his system to break out of his funk. Confronting him head-on was the only way to crack his hard exterior, win his respect, and get him to listen to me.

The irony is that he's way bigger than me. Colin's a kickboxer and I'm a skinny hippie. He could have beaten the shit out of me. But I knew what he needed to hear. Emotionally, he was behaving like a coward, and—for his own sake—he needed to snap out of it. I carried on. "You're hurting yourself and you're hurting her. I don't care if you want to hurt yourself, but stop hurting this woman."

Colin looked me in the eye and started crying. In a few moments, he was bawling his eyes out. "Thank you," he said. "I needed to hear that."

I told him that, after the retreat, he could tell her he loved her. Not because I said so, but because he genuinely felt it. I said, "That's what it means to be a masculine man. That's what it means to be a leader." He called his partner and said, "Baby, next time I see you, I've got something to tell you." Then he turned to me and said, "You know, if I left this retreat now, I'd be happy. I understand what I needed to get out of this."

The next time he and his partner had sex, it wasn't crazy, epic, throw-you-around-the-room shit. It was deep, slow, and emotionally connected. He told her he loved her, and they got to a new level of understanding and appreciation. Colin was amazed. He didn't realize that was an option. He started to see how he'd built up defenses against being controlled or manipulated because women had done that to him in the past, and he realized he could drop those defenses with his partner.

Colin understood that he didn't *always* need to try to be the man. He needed to connect with his gentleness. Sometimes, the best sex comes from looking into a woman's eyes, going slowly, and telling her how much you care about her.

After he left the retreat, Colin used this knowledge to become a better partner and father to his five kids, and he'll surely pass it on to his son in the future. He learned how to be real and understood that there are times when the most powerful thing a man can do is tell a woman he loves her.

If you want to know how to build deep emotional connections with women, go to sexualquantumleap.com/resources.

5

EVERY WOMAN IS DIFFERENT, EVERY PUSSY IS DIFFERENT

I met Eliza on Eliza Street in Adelaide, Australia. She was tall, brunette, and incredibly attractive, walking down the street toward me, wearing the sexiest boots I'd ever seen. Right away, I could tell she was something special. I knew I only had one chance to meet her and I wasn't going to pass it up.

"Are you lost?" I asked. Not the greatest opener, but it started a conversation. When she told me her name and I realized we were on Eliza Street, I decided it was destiny. We exchanged numbers and I texted her, asking what she was doing later that night. She told me she was busy with assignments and starting a new job the following day, but I persisted. Eventually, she agreed I could come over for a quick cup of tea around 12:30 a.m. that night. When we got together, the connection was electric.

When I looked into Eliza's eyes, I saw something deep and powerful and insanely sexy. That first night was off the hook. The next day, during her lunch break, she sent me a photo of her holding a banana, with the caption, "Please, sir, can I have some more?" I liked it.

We totally accepted each other, inside and outside the bedroom, and our next night together was even more electric. We both loved to play and explore, and we brought it out of each other. Pretty soon, we were hooked on each other and started dating. She lived in a beautiful cottage about two hundred meters from the beach. I live in Melbourne, so she used to fly down to visit or I would travel to stay at her place for five days at a time. Mostly, we just hung out, smoked weed, took drugs, and fucked.

Eliza really loved sex. She was supremely comfortable with her body and her desires. We were never bored, because we didn't hold anything back. Whatever we had to say, we said it, whether it was soft or raw. We shared lots of amazing nights, but there's one that really sticks out for me. We were throwing each other around, on the bed, on the kitchen counter, against the wall. It was very physical. At one point, she was on the bed while I choked her, kissed her, and played with her pussy.

I could tell she was about to squirt and, out of nowhere, something came to mind. I picked her off the bed, wrapped her legs around me, then stood her up and pinned her against the wall, one hand on her chest and the other inside her pussy. I could feel the pressure building up as I pleasured her, and her knees started to buckle. She'd already had loads of orgasms and I knew this was going to be the last one. She was ready to collapse and bask in the afterglow, but I leaned against her and held her upright with my arm and shoulder.

"I can't do any more!" she yelled. "Yes, you can!" I hollered back. "We'll do one more." She was losing her shit, squirting so much that there was a puddle on the floor underneath us, I reckon enough to half-fill a bucket. I was slipping in it, trying not to fall over. Her knees had completely given way. The only reason she was upright was because I was pressing her against the wall.

Eventually, her knees gave way and she sank to the floor. I pulled her slightly away from the wall and she lay on her back in her juices, while I continued to make her squirt. My knee was on her chest and she was panting, gripping my leg tightly in ecstasy. After we both caught our breath, I had a moment of inspiration. As she looked at me, as if to say, "What the fuck's going on?" I wedged one arm under her back and the other under her butt, picked her up, and started mopping up her juices with her hair.

"I fucking hate you!" she said. "It's going to take me like an hour and a half to wash my hair. But also, I fucking love you." People telling me they love me and hate me seems to be a theme of this book! Eliza did have the most amazing long, thick brown hair. She lay there, exhausted, covered in her own juices, exhausted from the orgasms and from being used as a human mop.

Why am I telling you this story? Because I'm a sick fuck? Yes, but also because I want you to understand that there are so many different ways to be sexual. This is an extreme example, used to illustrate not only how weird a sexual experience can be, but also how two people can totally welcome that, go with the flow, and have an amazing time together. This is true even when sex looks completely different from any expectations you might have picked up from the movies or porn, and when it goes against your perceptions of what you should do in the bedroom.

I'm not encouraging you to turn every woman you're with into a cleaning device. Far from it. All I'm saying is that Eliza and I gave each other permission to explore our desires. And they took us to a place that isn't in any textbook. It was fucking amazing.

You're probably thinking that you'd like to be able to turn a woman into a waterfall. The good news is, you can: go to sexualquantumleap.com/resources, and watch the squirting video.

THERE IS NO "ONE SIZE FITS ALL"

This chapter is about the reason why I don't *just* teach techniques. Guys come to me with the perception that if they learn the right techniques, they'll be "good" at sex. It doesn't work like that. Every woman is different, physically, psychologically, and emotionally. Something you did that made your ex cum might not have the same impact on a new woman.

I've been in open relationships and closed relationships. Both have their advantages and disadvantages. Eliza and I had an open relationship, which was both exciting and challenging. She was my main partner and I had two other partners in Melbourne. At the same time, I was dating other women casually. This time, I behaved ethically and everyone involved knew what was happening. Eliza was seeing an older man and another woman. I could write an entire book on dealing with the complex dynamics and the jealousy of open relationships. One time, we went to a sex party together. I was fucking her from behind while she went down on another woman, and I was fingering two chicks. Suddenly I felt a wave of love for her, stopped, and said, "Baby, I love you so much." The whole party stopped for a moment. She turned around and said, "I love you too, baby." Then everyone went back to what they were doing.

Some women would have found it impossible to feel fully expressed and comfortable in that context. But Eliza felt totally at home. The key to our sexual connection was allowing ourselves to explore. We didn't judge each other for our sexual expression. Instead, we consistently built each other up, making each other feel sexy and desirable, and allowing our naughty natures to shine through.

Let's be clear. What you need to do to please the woman in front of you might be completely different from any other woman you meet. Of course, there are similarities from one woman to the next. The basic anatomy is the same. But there are huge variations. Pussies are bigger and smaller, more and less sensitive. Some women have prominent labia, others not so much. Her body and the way she likes to be stimulated are unique.

Also, the woman you're with will be different at different points in her cycle. There will be times when she's not so interested in sex, others when she's really horny. When she's coming up to her period, she may feel bloated and totally unsexy. Her only desires may be for you to feed her chocolate, give her cuddles, rub her belly, put a hot water bottle on her tummy, and tell her she's pretty.

At any point in her cycle, she might be in a great mood, or she might have had a stressful day at work. Some days she'll want you to go slow and gentle. Other days she'll hunger to be pinned down and ravished. To truly be the best she's ever had, you need to get to know *her* individual body. Be willing to ask the hard questions and say the hard things.

Don't act like you know it all, and don't imagine that what worked with your last partner will definitely work with a new one. Truly get to know the woman in front of you. When you do that, she'll feel that you actually understand her body.

Most women won't come out and tell you if you're shit in bed. They're too polite. But you'll get indications, for sure. The universe first whispers, then speaks, then talks loudly, then finally screams, until you pay attention.

Don't wait until a woman is yelling at you, cheating on you, or leaving you. If she tells you more than once that she'd like to spend more time together, that's a good wake-up call. Think of it as a whisper from the universe. So many men think their women leave them, cheat on them, or lose interest in sex out of the blue. This is delusional. They have ignored the whispers and they're facing the consequences. Address the whispers and the universe won't need to scream at you.

To get genuine feedback from a woman, ask her simple questions. For example, invite her to tell you whether she wants you to go higher or lower, faster or slower, use more or less pressure. Those are simple, easy-to-follow directions that a woman can easily give you, even when she's so turned on she can hardly speak. Actual feedback from the woman you're with is the single best way to understand what she likes. It also feels great to her. If she says "slower" and you go slower, she will feel great knowing that you listened to her and did as she asked. As a result, she'll trust you more, and likely be more open to telling you much more about her sexuality.

Socrates' most famous saying, found in Plato's account of the philosopher, is "I know that I know nothing." Every time I'm with a woman, I adopt a beginner's mindset and remember that I know nothing. It's a great mindset to have when you're with a woman in the bedroom for the first time. She'll feel your humility, and that will enable her to relax.

Let her show you which parts of her pussy are most sensitive. You may know her G-spot from her clitoris, but there's so much variation. Some women need to be stimulated somewhere totally unique. For example, she may like it when you place pressure on certain parts of her body while you explore her pussy. Play, explore, and be messy. Be willing to ask the hard question and say the hard thing. Most importantly, don't expect to get everything right. This part of sex is definitely more art than science.

Sometimes people ask me who the hell I am to call myself a sex expert. The truth is, I'm not. I'm sure as hell not an academic or a clinical doctor, but I've got the street knowledge, the shit that actually matters. The only difference between me and the average guy is that I'm willing to admit how little I know. I go into a new experience wanting to understand the woman in front of me. How does her body work? What turns her on? I believe that's how a lot of amazing experiences happen.

EVERY WOMAN IS AN ANGEL AND A DEVIL

There are so many aspects to the female psyche. One thing's for sure, though; most women hide parts of themselves because they think they'll be judged harshly if they reveal them. There are individual differences, of course, but in general terms it's fair to say that every woman has a softer side and a wilder side.

When she's in her "angel," she'll want to be touched and caressed more gently. She'll prefer it if you move more slowly, with a focus on connection, so she can build a sense of safety. Don't rush it when she's in this mood. The last thing she'll want is the feeling that you're forcing things. Women hate the feeling that you are goal-orientated with a focus on reaching the point of orgasm. Instead, bring your attention to the moment, to your sensations and your breath.

At the other extreme, a woman's sexuality can be incredibly animalistic. She may want to be fucked roughly, held down, tied up, or have sex with multiple men. Women will only go to these places if they feel totally safe. It's as vulnerable for a woman to admit to her "devil" side as it is for her to snuggle up with you and melt into her "angel," and it can lead to just as much depth and connection.

I used to date a chick who, when she became totally comfortable with me, admitted that she fantasized about getting fucked by multiple guys. Although it wasn't a particular turn-on for me, I agreed to make that fantasy come true for her, and found the three hottest guys at a sex party we attended together—they looked like models. They went to town on her while I stood above her and fed her strawberries, and she called me "Daddy." She later decided that, although she was glad she did it, she wasn't too fussed about trying it again. When you encourage women to fully express their sexuality, you'll learn things about them that you could never have imagined and receive their gratitude and appreciation for inviting their full sexual expression.

Women who openly choose to have multiple sexual partners are often judged harshly and exposed to slut-shaming. Whatever you do, don't ever shame a woman for her sexuality. You'll shut her down immediately. If you sense that a woman is already shut down, discuss it with her. Ask her what's holding her back. Maybe she is struggling to come to terms with something from a past relationship.

You might wonder whether the woman you're with has the capacity to go to both of those extremes. She absolutely does, if she feels safe enough. That cute, shy girl you see in the coffee shop? Her devil side is in there, waiting for someone to uncover it. At the other end of the spectrum, a woman who's not had a lot of affection in her life might find it difficult to connect with her softer, angelic side, but it's there if you're willing to look hard enough for it. Me and my man Sim, AKA Black Mamba, had a wild night with a girl who adamantly refused to be cuddled after sex, until she eventually softened and said, "Fuck it, give me a cuddle."

Other women are at different stages. Maybe she was wild when she was younger and she's looking to explore a softer, slower sexual experience. Maybe she's always been a good girl and she wants to let her hair down. The only way you'll know for sure is by asking and exploring.

FOREPLAY IS EVERYTHING AND EVERYTHING IS FOREPLAY

You've likely heard the cliché that a man's a microwave and a woman's a slow cooker. For a woman, sex starts the moment she sees you. Everything from your body language to what you say when you open your mouth to talk to her for the first time is telling her a lot about you sexually. She's assessing what it's like to connect with you, and—by implication—what it would be like to have sex with you.

This isn't a book about meeting and attracting women, however, so let's assume that you've got a woman to the point where she's at least willing to kiss you. Take your time and establish presence, using lots of eye contact. The lips are full of nerve endings and a good kissing experience can go from being slow and sensual to more powerful and assertive. I've never met a woman who doesn't enjoy kissing, and every woman I've asked appreciates it when a man kisses her with full presence, not as though he's doing it just to get to the sex part.

Years ago, I got an education in this experience. I was at a conscious sex party for hippies called a "sacred temple," and a woman who told me she was a goddess looked at me and said, "Kiss me with absolute presence." At the time, the idea was alien to me. I looked at her a bit sarcastically. But I did it. And it was amazing. I was totally concentrated on the experience of her lips meeting mine. Nothing else. There's no need to dictate a rhythm when you kiss. Get lost in the moment and find the mutual rhythm. Let your lips and tongue dance with hers, matching her tempo and embracing the flow between you.

Another thing you can do during foreplay is give her back tickles. Run your hands over her back, gently at first, then maybe with more pressure. If she's into it, you can use your nails and give her some scratches. It's a very relaxing motion, which should allow her to drop into her body and relax. In time, that relaxation will become a turn-on. But don't rush it. Don't reach for her pussy too early. Just enjoy giving the back tickles.

Caress her face, from her forehead down to her chin. Like the back tickles, it's a very nurturing form of touch that breeds a deep sense of safety. It's a very nurturing, caring sensation. Give great hugs. Pull her in close so she can feel that you've got her. Allow her to let go. No pressure, just the warmth and safety of holding her in your arms. If necessary, tell her explicitly to relax, take her time, and enjoy the moment. Buying a massage table and learning a few basics never hurts, either.

Another way to build sexual tension is with messages. Tell her you've been thinking about her and how sexy she is, text her what you want to do with her, let her know you can't wait for the next time you see each other. Little things like that will keep you on her mind, so she'll anticipate the next time you see each other. Turn your texting into a miniature erotic novel. Try sending her a photo of yourself in nothing but a towel, just after you step out of the shower, or right after you finish a workout at the gym. "Just got out of the shower, thinking of you ;)" or "Just finished a workout, thinking of you ;)." These are great messages for women you have recently started seeing, especially when you know you're meeting up later that day or week. This has the added bonus of being a great way to start a text exchange of naughty photos. Go on, show her the cannons!

Finally, remember that sex is so much more than cock in pussy. It's so much more than an outcome. It's an experience to share. The pussy isn't the main course. It's dessert. Take your time getting there and enjoy the buildup. If you already think you're going slowly, slow down even more. Tease her until she's begging *you* to speed up. Have the discipline not to enter her until she's desperate for you to fuck her. To the point where she's borderline annoyed with you because she wants you inside her so badly. She may be slightly irritated in the moment, but her orgasms will be so much better because you truly got her ready. In case you need a reminder of how to do this, reread the section on dominance!

Most women are constantly distracted by things they think they should be doing. "I need to feed the dog. I need to check Facebook. I need to get back to work." Foreplay is a way to bring her out of her mind, into her body and the present moment with you, so she can relax enough to get deeply turned on. If a woman isn't present with you in bed, it's terrible. You will absolutely feel it. To become a master at building sexual tension, take the training at sexualquantumleap.com/resources.

SEXUAL EXPRESSION

This is what a lot of people would call dirty talk. I don't really like the phrase; I prefer "sexual expression." To call something "dirty" implies that it's wrong. Even the phrases "blow job" and "hand job" sound like work, not like amazing experiences to share.

What turns you on verbally? Things you say, things she says? What do you want to say to her inside the bedroom? Now, what do *you* like her to say to you? In what tone of voice? How do you want her to look at you while she says it?

If you're seeing someone, have you asked her what she likes to hear from you in the bedroom? What does she like you to call her, for example? Is there anything she really *doesn't* want you to call her? Maybe she loves it when you tell her she's a dirty slut. Maybe she's not into that at all. Calibrate with her and find out. I used to love calling an ex-girlfriend of mine an "Asian hooker," but she hated it, so I agreed to stop.

Sexual expression doesn't have to be dirty. It can be beautiful and uplifting. You can tell her how much you like and appreciate her, or how much you love her, if that's true. You can even extend it outside the bedroom, using the same principles. What do you want her to say to you? What does she need you to say to feel loved, nourished, and appreciated? What words and tone does she want you to use for maximum impact?

When you're on your own, you can look in the mirror and practice what you want to say, then check in with your partner and ask her whether she likes it. At other times, something might come up spontaneously while you're together. As long as it's not something she's asked you not to say to her, feel free to express it.

So many guys are silent in the bedroom. They may be talkative in other situations, but in their most intimate moments, they stop talking. Why do that? There are so many ways to express yourself. It doesn't have to feel dirty. You can tell her what you appreciate about her body or share a sexual fantasy. You can tell her how much you care about her. Whatever it is, let it come through you.

THREE STAGES OF FEMALE ORGASM

Although we've talked about every woman being different, there are similarities. The process of reaching an orgasm is generally similar. Every woman can have multiple orgasms. The hardest thing for many is allowing themselves to surrender fully.

Some women have a religious background and have been told that they shouldn't touch themselves or have sex before marriage. They may be anxious about receiving pleasure and start to judge themselves. Others feel like they need to place an extremely high value on their sexuality. Still others may feel uncomfortable and need more reassurance before they're ready to relax.

If a woman isn't psychologically ready to cum, she won't cum. Your manhood isn't based on how many orgasms you give her. If she feels that you are trying to force her to cum, she certainly won't. It's not your job to make a woman cum. It's her job to bring herself into that state. It's her job to understand her body and know what brings her pleasure. But you can help.

Women from different backgrounds will have different attitudes to pleasure and relationships. You'll want to select a woman whose values match your own. Choose your partners based on your desired experiences.

Stage One: Letting Go

Letting go comes from feeling that she can trust you, that you have her best interests at heart, and that you're not going to judge her. Most guys try to leap ahead to the orgasm itself, but that's not going to work. Fundamentally, you need a woman to let go before she's ready to orgasm.

Don't judge your performance in bed purely on whether a woman cums. For some women, letting go and feeling genuine pleasure may be a huge breakthrough. If you want some feedback, resist the temptation to seek validation. Instead, come from a place of curiosity. "How was that experience for you?" is more inviting than, "Did you cum?" It will open up the space for her to tell you honestly what she enjoyed and what she'd like to do differently. If you're genuinely curious about whether she came, ask because you want to understand her experience and learn what she'd like you to do differently next time, not because you're seeking validation or to suggest that there's something wrong if she didn't. Fundamentally, this stage is about inviting a woman to open up and feel deeply relaxed, creating the potential for orgasm. When she is relaxed, she can cum. When she feels stressed or pressured, she won't.

Women who aren't used to letting go may even think that they have had an orgasm just because they feel so relaxed. If a woman is unsure whether she has cum, but knows it felt great, it probably means she's allowed herself to get out of her head and into her body for the first time in a while.

Stage Two: One Orgasm

When a woman feels that you're not pressuring her to cum, and you're not in a hurry to get anywhere then, paradoxically, she's more likely to cum. Let her know that it's okay for her not to cum, that you're cool with playing, relaxing, and exploring, and you'll likely heighten her pleasure. When she's really relaxed and enjoying herself, her body and mind will open up to orgasm.

If she's not ready to cum from your touch, or if you want to try something fun and different, ask her to show you how she pleasures herself. Some women like to put a pillow between their legs or lay on their side. Others like to be on their front. Some squeeze a certain part of their body. Some women need lots of pressure on their clit or G-spot, whereas some women need barely any pressure. Be curious. If a woman shows you something unusual, take an interest and feel relaxed excitement. She probably doesn't show many people. You can also try masturbating next to each other, so you get really turned on.

Stage Three: Multiple Orgasms

When a woman gets fully comfortable with you and with herself, she can move into multiple orgasms. This is stage three. At this point, she's so relaxed that she lets go and gives herself permission to surrender herself to you. She keeps cumming, over and over again. It's a powerful and humbling experience. Encourage this by constantly letting her know how much you love seeing her in pleasure.

More than an orgasm—or multiple orgasms—a woman wants a place to let go and be all of who she is sexually. Some women judge themselves so harshly. When you can create a space that allows her to get out of her head, into her body, and forget about self-judgment, she will thank you. Remember breath, sound, movement, and vocal expression (BSMV)? Encourage her BSMV. This is the best way for her to experience as much presence and pleasure as possible.

THE SIX S'S OF SEXUALITY

The Six S's of Sexuality is a concept I've discovered and developed over the past few years, as I've started to break down sex, relationships, and the mechanics of connection. If you can hit all six of these, you'll blow a woman's mind in the bedroom, to the point where you may get more female attention than you know how to handle.

As we've discussed, every woman is different. But there are some common principles you can apply to your interactions with women. We've talked about several of them already, and this is a great way to put them all together. Use these Six S's wisely.

One: Safe

This is the first and most important component of the Six S's, which is why it comes first. If a woman doesn't feel safe with you, there is zero chance she will be able to relax, let go, and open herself up to pleasure. Can she open up with you? Can she tell you her deepest desires and trust that you'll respect them? The key to safety is consent. Whatever you want to do, do it with consent. If you don't have consent, don't go there.

To make a woman feel safe, work on the foundations of trust between the two of you. When she knows and trusts you, you will gain her respect. The deeper her trust and respect, the more she will feel safe and let go, completely giving herself over to pleasure.

The best way to build trust is to encourage open, honest conversations where any topic can be freely discussed. Ask her questions no other man has asked her, because you want to understand her desires, needs, and anxieties, and the reasons she feels this way. She wants to know that you accept her, that you're curious about her sexuality, and that you have her best interests at heart.

Your goal here is to create a space in which she can be her real, authentic sexual self with you, where she feels so comfortable that she's willing to tell you anything and everything about her sexuality, including things she has never dared to share with other men. No matter what she says, remember to accept her sexuality. Under no circumstances should you start judging her. If a woman feels that you're looking at her through judgmental eyes, she will stop feeling safe and shut down, a principle that applies both inside and outside the bedroom.

Two: Seen

We all long to be seen for who we are, including our flaws and imperfections. Can you see a woman in her full humanity, and take an interest in the person she is? I'm not just talking about her body here. Are you interested in the depths of her soul? A woman wants you to look beyond the mask she puts on and perceive the parts of her she doesn't allow the world to see. She wants you to notice her insecurities and the walls she puts up. She wants to feel that you know who she is behind all the complexities, and that you love her anyway.

There is a simple rule you can follow to help women achieve the most intense orgasms: unlock her mind and her body will follow. In simple terms, the more deeply you get to know who she is at her core, the better the orgasms will be for both of you. The only way to get to know her at this deep level is to ask her precise, specific questions. Aim to get to know her better than any other man. Ask her questions most people wouldn't think to ask. Ask the hard questions that no man *wants* to ask, and also learn to say the hard things that no man wants to say.

Once this practice becomes a natural part of the way you relate to women, you will be on the path toward fully seeing and understanding the core of any woman you are with. When you see her for who she is, she'll be excited to show you more of herself. It's easy to have sex without engaging emotionally. It's much harder to open up her mind and heart so that she feels totally seen.

Three: Sexy

The third S is sexy. Ensure that the woman you're with knows that you find her irresistibly sexy. She wants to feel your passion and desire for her emanating from your body. She wants to feel unique and special, and confident that you find her sexy in ways that other men never have. She wants you to feel her, desire her, and to allow your fiery passion for her to overrule caution.

Your goal here is to make her feel like the most desired woman on the planet. Animals are basic and instinctual creatures. They see what they want, and they take it. For most women, receiving this kind of desire is a huge fantasy. When you're with a woman sexually, let your inner animal shine through. Trust that she wants to feel your sexual presence and insatiable desire, rooted in love and care.

When you show a woman your desire for her, she'll feel sexy. That can be a pulsing, animalistic hunger, or it can be a subtle glance of affection and lust. You can let a woman know that you find her sexy by ripping her clothes off and ravishing her body, or by commenting on how much you appreciate some small aspect of her clothes or makeup. The vibe here is that you're so attracted to her that you can't help but want to take her and deeply ravish her.

Send her sexy messages. Let her know what turns you on about her. You can be really specific. Do you love the way she's done her hair today? Is there a particular dress she wears that turns you on?

Women love this kind of confidence. When you show up authentically, unafraid of expressing how you truly feel in the moment, she will feel your passion. When she knows that what you say is rooted in your desire for her, she will absolutely feel like the center of your desire. When you do this, you can keep her feeling sexy and deeply desired even years into a relationship.

Four: Scared

Scared? What the fuck? This is the most controversial aspect of the Six S's, and for good reason. It confuses a lot of people. You might be wondering, "Why would I want her to be scared of me?" In this context, however, what I mean by "scared" is that you want her to feel your raw masculine power. She wants to know, deep in her bones, that you can take her and ravish her.

Obviously, I'm not saying that your woman should be outright terrified of you. Far from it. I'm saying that she should feel your strength and know that there's a primal element to your being, just below the surface—and sometimes breaking through the surface.

She also wants to trust that you know your own mind, that you respect your own boundaries, and that you can stand up strongly for what you believe when called. In a word, she wants to know that you can dominate her. She wants to submit to you, let go, and follow your lead. She wants to feel the thrill of knowing that you're in your power, that you know how to protect her, and that you can lead her where you want to go. A woman can't love you unless she respects you and a woman will respect you when you take control, know what you want, and go for it.

Like many of my clients, you may be fearful of your capacity for dominance. Maybe you don't trust yourself to unleash the beast within because you're afraid of hurting your woman—if so, try out for the wrestling exercise from the previous chapter. Remember, you are coming from a place of wanting the best for her, not wishing to do her harm. She should understand that you would never use your strength to hurt her, but at the same time, there's an unpredictability to you. She can't control you. She never knows when you might pin her down and over-power her. That's an exhilarating feeling for a woman.

Five: Sexual

Yeah, we're including both sexy and sexual in the Six S's. This is a book about sex, after all. For a woman to feel relaxed and comfortable with you sexually, she needs to know that you are comfortable with your own sexuality. Being sexual is about understanding what you like, and what sexual experiences you want to explore. Once you know what turns you on and you're comfortable with your own sexual expression, you can begin to ask for what you want and explore new frontiers with a woman.

The point here is that she needs to perceive you as a sexual man: someone who's confident and at ease with his sexuality. Women are highly intuitive. When you are sexually open, she'll know. Likewise, she will know when you are holding back or out of touch with your sexuality. If you are struggling to express yourself in this area, however, don't worry. It's totally possible to become increasingly comfortable with your sexuality, as I hope you've already realized from reading this book!

Most of us men keep this side of ourselves bottled up, in a misguided effort to protect our partners. This will always lead to relationship dysfunction, potential cheating, neglect, and feelings of misunderstanding. You like it when a woman opens up to you, right? By the same token, if she's into you, she'll like it when you open up to her. Can you sit in your desire, enjoy it for what it is, without feeling a need to instantly relieve the tension? Can you share what you like with a woman?

You need to lead by going first and expressing what you need and want. This will give her permission to be open about her own sexuality in turn. The more you do this together, the more you will create a deeper bond. Sex isn't dirty and taboo. It is beautiful. The more comfortable you are being a sexual man, the more you'll magnetize women to you.

Six: Soft

Finally, let's talk about softness. This is the gentleness we've discussed in previous chapters. Do you know how to move slowly, appreciate each moment, and forget about the destination?

You've read about how a woman wants to be pinned down, ravished, and fucked hard, which is absolutely true. But that is only one aspect of sexuality. Women also desire gentle and soft lovemaking. A woman wants someone who makes her feel cared for, loved, and appreciated. Bring out a woman's softness with back tickles; slow, deep kisses; and taking your time to explore her body. Dance together to slow, gentle music. Tell her how much you care about her. These are the things that will allow her to melt into softness.

As a man, I know bringing softness can be one of the hardest parts of this guide. Societal pressure leads us to believe that being a man means hiding our emotions and hardening up. This is an extremely toxic way to live, which leads men to build up their walls and allow negativity to fester inside them. Your partner should be one person you feel safe with, and with whom you open up and express yourself fully.

This step can be especially hard for highly ambitious men who try hard to deny their emotions. If you're not comfortable with your emotions, however, she will feel that you're not comfortable with her emotions either. In time, she'll feel that you neglect her.

Your woman wants to be part of your life, including the good, the bad, and the ugly. She wants to be by your side through your successes and failures, cheering you on when you knock it out of the park and picking you back up when you have a bad day. It can be tough opening up and expressing vulnerability, but we're all human. We all feel vulnerable sometimes. When you own it, you'll be able to share a lot more pleasure.

APPRECIATE HER UNIQUENESS

When you truly understand a woman's body and her pleasure, you will see her in a different light. You'll appreciate what makes her unique and you'll unlock her body in ways she's never known before.

When you can do this for a woman, don't be surprised if she's grateful to you for being in her life and bringing her so much pleasure. Most women struggle to find a place where they can be fully expressed and feel huge appreciation for a man who can create that environment.

It's extremely satisfying to watch a woman blossom into the best possible version of herself sexually. Few men know how to support this process, so when you do, you'll be rare and in demand. I want you to feel as though you're celebrating her sexuality and the woman she is.

That may lead you to some weird and wonderful places. My experiences with Eliza aren't a template for you to follow. They're an illustration of one direction sexuality can go. Sex is an art and a science. There are underlying principles, but there's also an element of it that can only take place in the moment, responding to her desires and yours as they become clear.

When you know how to combine technique and heart, you'll be unstoppable. My experience with Eliza was about constantly diving into the unknown and discovering what was there for us to explore. It was a celebration of her sexuality and mine. We never felt that our sexual expression had to look a certain way. We just danced with it. As a result, our connection kept getting better and better.

It's important to understand the principles behind sexuality, but equally, be willing to drop your ideas of how sex is supposed to look. How can you be as free as possible? How can you give yourself permission to be fully expressed? How can you create the sexual experiences you crave?

Don't try to be like me. Don't try to emulate your favorite porn star. Be like you. Allow your natural expression to shine through.

6

PRACTICAL WAYS TO BOOST YOUR SEX LIFE

Lusty came from a traditional Italian family. Mama and Nona ruled his life, and he was convinced that it was his destiny to meet a good Italian woman who would cook great pasta and be a mother to his children. Just the idea of diverging from that path made him break out in a cold sweat.

He was also quite overweight—probably from eating all that pasta. At five feet, five inches, Lusty weighed 110 kilos (242 pounds). Sexually, Lusty's self-esteem was at the bottom of the ocean. He was fat, addicted to porn, and if he ever did get naked with a woman, he came so fast it was over before it had properly begun.

Weirdly, however, he had a huge ego. We met at a dating event and he insisted on telling me about his conquests. At first, I thought he was a weird guy, but he was a videographer and I needed someone to do some filming for me. Back then,

I didn't have the money to hire a videographer, so I took the chance to find one where I could. We made a deal: I'd help him with women, and he'd film some videos for my website. "Stick with me," I told him, "and I promise you'll have the wildest sexual experiences of your life, and a dating life you can only dream of right now."

He wasn't sure whether I was the real deal, but he believed me enough to give it a try. With all his family and religious conditioning about sexuality, I could see I had an uphill battle in front of me, but I figured, "Fuck it. What have I got to lose?"

I started by telling him some painful home truths. "You're fat," I said. "You need to lose a lot of weight. You hang out with shitty people and you've got a bad fucking attitude." That level of directness hit him like a ton of bricks. "You're right, man," he replied. "Thank you." That level of authenticity became the foundation of one of my best friendships.

With Lusty, we were starting from scratch. He had very little experience with women, having attended an all-boys school. I took him out with me to meet women, both during the day and at night; at first, he was terrified. He kept wanting to stay at home, watch porn, and play video games instead of coming out and meeting women. He hated the idea of failing, but he equally hated the idea of taking a woman home and struggling with premature ejaculation. I saw him break down in tears on multiple occasions, convinced that he'd never enjoy the connections he craved with women.

In the end, Lusty conquered his demons. He lost about thirty-five kilos (seventy-seven pounds) and got in good shape. We became gym buddies, and I was in the best shape of my life too. His confidence improved and he felt comfortable meeting women anywhere, from coffee shops to clubs. He found a girlfriend who respected him, which ironically brought a whole new set of challenges. How would he respond to the temptations of other women?

Lusty broke through a lot of social conditioning. At first, he wasn't interested in using sex toys. He just wanted to have "normal" sex. Over time, he got comfortable playing with every toy imaginable. He ended up shooting some porn with us and laughing about it later. "Never in my wildest dreams, man," he said, "did I imagine that I'd be doing this." He came a long way from the shy, fat guy who could hardly talk to a woman.

PRACTICAL ADVICE AND IDEAS

This chapter is full of practical tips. You'll find a ton of exercises to turn you into an absolute boss in the bedroom, such as the Seven Nights of Sin. Plus, if you're struggling with performance anxiety, premature ejaculation, or erectile dysfunction, you'll find focused help here.

We're going from theory to takeaways you can apply to your real life to get real results. As with the material in the previous chapter, I've held it back until this part of the book because I wanted you to have the foundations before you dive into the more practical elements of improving your sex life. It's important that you know yourself and your partner, rather than thinking that these ideas will automatically sort out any problems with your sex life.

If all you wanted was technique, you could have picked up any number of other books, so I trust that you've stayed with me up to this point. The foundations we have laid will allow you to make the most out of the ideas in this chapter.

Once you've mastered the techniques in this part of the book, you'll feel more comfortable with your sexuality. If you know you're not going to struggle with premature ejaculation or erectile dysfunction, it's so much easier to get out of your head and enjoy the moment. That'll have an impact on how you relate to women, inside and outside the bedroom.

Use the concepts you've learned throughout this book and apply them to the exercises in this chapter. Then, get feedback from your partner—and also from yourself. What did you like? What would you do differently? The more you iterate, the more you'll learn. Some of the exercises in this chapter may seem weird or silly at first. Trust me, there's a method to the madness, honed by me and thousands of clients around the world. When you get comfortable being uncomfortable, you'll build so much confidence in your physical expression. Give the ideas in this chapter a try. What have you got to lose?

A NOTE ON PHYSICAL, MENTAL, AND EMOTIONAL HEALTH

This isn't a book about diet and exercise, or even about mental and emotional health—although we definitely touch on those elements of sex. I could talk for hours about the influence of those factors on your sexuality, but this book isn't the right place.

Nonetheless I want to give you a very brief overview of the mental, emotional, and physical aspects of PE and ED, and offer a few pointers for your further research. Some people will tell you that performance issues are purely physical. Others will say they're a mental issue. Still others will point to the emotional aspect of sex. In fact, performance issues are a combination of all three. The mind, body, and emotions are all linked. To maintain rock-hard erections all night, you need to handle all three.

Mental

If your mind is troubled, how will you be present with a woman? Stress and anxiety will increase the risk of performance issues. If you experience critical self-talk about your sexuality, and struggle to quiet your mind, you need to do something about it. Perhaps you're holding on to stories about your sexuality, or lost in thoughts of the past, present, or future. All of that will make it much harder for you to relax and be present.

The good news is that there are lots of ways to calm your mind and bring yourself into the present moment, so you can focus on the good stuff—like the woman in front of you. Awareness is the first step. Then you need to unlock the stories and loops in your mind that keep you from being present. Way back in Chapter One, we talked about changing your sexual story. If you're struggling with PE and ED, revisit that exercise. Ask yourself about your connection to sexuality. Are you so caught up trying to perform that you can't relax and enjoy yourself? Are you being honest with yourself and the woman in front of you about your wants, desires, and boundaries?

To quiet the mind prior to sex, try closing your eyes and taking some deep belly breaths to quiet the mind. As thoughts arise, allow them to pass away. Alternatively, try meditating on the stories you are telling yourself about your sexuality. Practice these techniques for ten minutes, or as long as you feel comfortable. Meditation is tremendous for psychological relaxation. It can help you to become present and prevent your thoughts from running rampant.

Emotional

The mind and emotions are linked, so there's a lot of overlap between this section and the previous one, although the focus here is more on your emotional experience, as opposed to your mental processes.

If you have a negative perception of your sexuality, you'll find it difficult to get turned on when you're with a woman. Maybe there have been moments in your life when you've experienced sexual pain and, as a result, shut down. Many of the men I work with fear opening up emotionally. Others get anxious about being too rough in the bedroom. Sometimes both.

Often, the root of these issues is sexual shame or guilt. If you struggle with sexual shame, you need to uncover and release those emotions; otherwise you'll bring them into the bedroom and they'll disrupt your experience, just when you want to be relaxing and feeling into your sensations. Only you really know your emotions; it's up to you to find a way of exploring, naming, and releasing any that are holding you back.

For a lasting effect, you may need to dive deeply into your psyche and discover what's driving your negative emotions. Neuro-linguistic programming (NLP), hypnosis (either with a therapist or using audio, or both), or cognitive behavioral therapy (CBT) may help you to unravel your sexual stories and related emotions. A regular meditation practice can also be helpful in releasing emotions, as can different forms of breathwork, such as Wim Hof breathing.

Physical

I'm not here to fat-shame, but the simple fact is that if you're significantly overweight, it will have an impact on your sexual performance. Exercise, especially exercises of the pelvis, improves blood flow throughout the body, while resistance training boosts testosterone. From a sexual perspective, both are good things. Hiking, sprints, and full-body calisthenic movements also strengthen and tone the body. On retreats, we teach specific exercises such as the five Tibetan rites of rejuvenation, which build strength and vitality. In Eastern philosophy, these exercises are known as the fountain of youth. Gratitude to Tao for teaching them to me.

There's lots of information on the internet about specific foods that have a positive impact on libido, so I won't dwell long on them here. Grass-fed beef, for example, is believed to improve the male hormone profile. Ashwagandha, shilajit, shatavari, and Aphro-D are supplements renowned for their effects on male sexuality. Asparagus leads to bigger loads, while oysters—in fact, any shellfish—are powerful aids to male sexual health. The basic principles are simple: eat healthy wild-caught or gathered or hunted foods and you'll see an upturn in your sex drive. Finally, stay away from sugars and processed foods, which tank your libido.

There is way more to say about this subject than I can cover in this book. For a deeper dive on getting PE and ED handled, take a trip to sexualquantumleap.com/resources.

THINK ABOUT CONNECTION BEFORE PERFORMANCE

Here's the horrible reality for a lot of guys. Like Lusty, they sabotage potential connections because they're full of anxiety about what could go wrong. Instead of breathing into that anxiety, they go into performance mode to try and cover up their emotions. They worry about cumming too quickly, not cumming at all, or whether they'll get it up and keep it up. If they go on dates, they choose women who are below their standards, to lower the stakes. That means they have less connection and less meaning in their lives. If they have a partner, they shy away from the deep, real conversations that bring aliveness, meaning, and connection.

The truth is that the kind of women you want to keep in your life respect honesty. If you cum too quickly or can't get it up, a cool woman will be understanding. She wants you to relax and enjoy yourself.

You can even put it on the table and say, "Hey, sometimes when I'm with someone for the first time, I need a little time to relax. Let's have a bath and chill for a while." It's okay to cuddle or play around. It's okay to take the pressure off yourself. Don't succumb to the idea that, as a man, you have to be rock-hard on command. Maybe your sexuality isn't so much like a microwave after all. Maybe you too are more like a slow cooker, taking time to warm up. That is completely fine.

You might be thinking, "Yeah, that's alright for you to say, Andrew. You don't have any problems." Believe me, I know what it's like. I also put myself under a lot of pressure, because I'm out there as the guy who teaches men how to be the best she's ever had. I get women reaching out to me expecting me to be incredible in bed. Yeah, I know, it's a hard life.

I give myself permission to take that pressure away, to focus on presence before performance. It's easy to be seduced by pills, sprays, and creams, but your cock will respond to how relaxed and connected you are with the person in front of you.

To encourage that connection, never force yourself to make shit happen. Allow and welcome your body's authentic responses, connect to your emotions, and express what's on your mind. It helps tremendously.

I've been in multiple situations where I couldn't get it up or came too quickly. Every time I admit to a woman that I'm a bit nervous, I feel better. Some guys might perceive that as weakness, but most women really appreciate it. On the few occasions where women haven't been cool, they're people I don't want in my life.

Take the pressure off yourself and realize that sex doesn't have to be amazing every time, especially not the first night. If you sometimes lose your erection, that's normal. You're only human. This goes double if you've recently been through a breakup and you still feel an emotional link with your ex. Nonetheless, whenever I connect my head, heart, and cock, I relax and open up. In those circumstances, I've never had a problem getting hard or cumming too quickly.

EXERCISES FOR SEXUAL MASTERY

Alright, here goes. Exercises you can explore to deepen your relationship with your sexuality and improve your connection with a partner. We'll start with things you can do alone, then move on to practices you can do with a partner.

Penis Appreciation

The first step to sexual mastery is mastering your relationship with your sword. What do you think of your penis? So many guys feel shame and guilt about it. There's no need to feel that way. Your cock's amazing, and an important part of who you are. Take some time to appreciate it.

This exercise is simple and profound. Place your hands over your cock and balls, breathe deeply, and observe what comes up. What happens? Do you start to feel nervous? Do your hands get sweaty? Do you find yourself hunching over?

The reaction might not be negative. Maybe you'll feel great. Whatever happens physiologically, welcome it. Verbally appreciate your genitals by saying something like, "Thank you for being an integral part of my life. You're important to me. Thank you for all the experiences we've had together." Give your cock and balls whatever positive affirmations you want.

Before doing this exercise, most guys think it's the weirdest thing they'll ever do. Afterward, they think it's the best. When you appreciate your penis, women will start to appreciate it as well. It's a part of who you are. The more you're rooted in appreciation of it, the more women will feel and enjoy your sexual presence.

Sadly, many men feel like their sexuality is worthless. They think that women are doing them a favor by having sex with them. They don't believe that they *deserve* to have great sex. This kind of appreciation exercise is a great reminder that your part in sex is indispensable. It's a way to build positive associations with your sexuality, and to remind yourself that you and your cock are friends, not foes. We have a dedicated training on penis appreciation at sexualquantumleap.com/resources.

Fuck Her in the Heart

This exercise builds on the penis appreciation one. To take it to the next level, see your penis as an extension of your heart. When you penetrate a woman sexually, you penetrate her with love. See your cock as a wand of light, and visualize yourself using it to love, liberate, and empower women you have sex with.

This is a great way to banish shame and solidify your sense of your penis as a force for good. This will allow you to relax into your sexuality and see it as a loving part of you. Plus, women will feel so much more connected to you. For a guided meditation on fucking her in the heart, go to—you guessed it—sexualquantumleap.com/resources.

Seduce Yourself

One of the most common problems I see with guys is that they feel stuck in their physical sexual expression. They don't know how to move freely or respond in the moment. This is exacerbated by a culture that admires stiff, highly built male bodies.

To feel free in the bedroom, you need to feel free in your body. That means you need to move unselfconsciously. Fortunately, I have a weird exercise to get you out of your head and into pleasurable physical expression. Like the penis appreciation, this one seems super weird and embarrassing to most guys before they try it. But it's an amazing way to cut through anxiety.

When you're alone, put on a slow, sexy song, and start dancing to it, seducing yourself in the mirror. Move your body slowly and sensually. At first, you may feel awkward as hell. Most guys are locked in the hips and find it hard to gyrate in a way that feels sexy.

As you open up and start moving, feel free to run your hands over your body. Express yourself with breath, sound, movement, and vocal expression. You'll find that you begin to feel the music and drop into a rhythm. There's no outcome you need to reach, nowhere to get to. Just you and the music.

For the intermediate experience, take your clothes off and do this dance naked. For some real next-level shit, do it in front of a woman. Dancing slowly and sexily in front of a woman is pretty confronting. But it brings great confidence. You don't need to have amazing stripper moves. Just hold eye contact, move, and let go. You'll get so much more comfortable in your body, which will translate to amazing sexual presence. Watch how turned on she gets, but stay present to your own movement.

You can do this practice every day. To make it even more powerful, combine it with an animal dance. This is the same idea, but instead of dancing slowly and sensually, you go totally wild. Jump around like crazy, scream and shout like a monkey, or channel your wild animal warrior energy. Move your body in any way that feels natural. Whatever you want to express, let it out.

After you've tried both the soft version and the animalistic version, reflect on them. Which one felt easier and more comfortable? Where did you struggle or feel self-conscious? Practice transitioning between the two energies.

A Deeper Level of Self-Pleasure

Most guys use self-pleasure as a way to get a quick release. It feels good, but they're training themselves to concentrate their pleasure in their genitals and to cum quickly. It's possible to feel pleasure all over your body. If you struggle with premature ejaculation, this is a great way to build pleasure up more slowly, rather than going for the orgasm in a couple of minutes. Your whole body is an erogenous zone, not just your cock and balls. We need to wake up the nerve endings!

There are four stages of self-pleasure to explore. I highly recommend that you take the time to fully experience all of them.

Stage One: Solo, without touching your genitals.

It's a really good idea to get familiar with your body *without* going for your cock. Take your time. Set the mood with some music. Caress your entire body. How does it feel to touch your chest, your legs, your arms? Don't judge the sensations, just feel them. Try rubbing oil on your body: sesame oil for a warming effect or coconut oil for a cooling sensation. This will condition you to enjoy all sorts of sensations, not just genital touch.

Stage Two: Solo, including your genitals.

Naturally, this is the next stage. Get comfortable in the bath, shower, or on your bed. When you're ready to touch your genitals, keep the movement slow. Explore the whole area. If you don't get hard straightaway, that's cool. Just enjoy the sexual pleasure circling throughout your body. Don't rush to give yourself maximum stimulation.

Stage Three: Receiving from a partner.

This moves masturbation from a solo practice to a partner practice, but it follows naturally from the previous exercises, so let's go with it. When you're with a woman, ask her to rub coconut oil over and massage your entire body. Allow yourself to relax into the sensations throughout your body. You might think women won't be into this, but you'd be surprised. If you've learned anything from this book, I hope it's that many women are fully open to exploring all kinds of sexual experiences when they feel your openness. Sometimes, it is super challenging to receive. Then you can do the same for her another time to allow her to receive. Sometimes women find it hard to receive and let go so this will be a treat for her.

Stage Four: Self-pleasure together.

Lying in bed masturbating together is a great way to feel seen, discover what your partner likes, and share a hot, sensual experience. It's also an amazing way to get turned on without going straight for the orgasm. All of these stages will help you build up sensation in your body, without blowing your load at the earliest moment. Build it up and edge together, get to the point of no return, and back it off then build it up again. Play the game of seeing who can resist touching the other person for the longest.

BRINGING A PARTNER INTO YOUR LIFE

If you don't already have a partner, consciously choose your next. You probably already know that vision work can be incredibly powerful. When you see something in your mind's eye, you can imagine making it happen. To call the perfect partner into your life, imagine them first, in great detail.

Start by creating an environment that helps you to connect with your desires. Close your eyes and imagine your perfect partner. What does she look like? How does it feel to be with her? What does she value in life? Imagine her personality. Is she bubbly? Passionate? Affectionate? What qualities do you see in her?

What does she like to do? Is she into dancing? Does she prefer to chill in front of a movie? Is she active? What are her hobbies and interests? How about her sexual personality? What's she into? What would you love to explore with her?

Write down everything you want to do with her and all the things you want to say to her. What would your perfect day together look like? Your perfect sexual experience? We'll touch on doing this with a partner later in the chapter, but you can also do it alone. When you do meet a partner, you'll have a head start. You can let her know that you've already done this exercise and invite her to do the same.

THE PERFECT PARTNER MEDITATION

This exercise works whether you're single or partnered. It's about discovering your fullest sexual expression. As men, we often try to please the woman in front of us. By connecting deeply with our sexuality when there's no woman present, we can break out of this habit and focus on our own desires, which in turn is highly erotic for women.

Find somewhere you can be alone and feel comfortable expressing yourself as loudly as you want. The bedroom's an obvious choice. Start by placing one hand on your heart and the other on your cock and balls, or both on your cock and balls if that feels more comfortable. I recommend choosing three different songs: one soft and gentle, representing the sensual seductress; the second harder and rougher, representing the masculine warrior; and the third freestyle. You can also decide to practice just one mood for as long as you want on any given day. With your eyes closed and the music you've selected playing, start moving your body. Pretend that you're making love to your perfect partner, whether she's someone you haven't met yet or you're already in a relationship with her. Picture her right there in front of you. Give yourself fully to the visceral experience. Do the things you've always wanted to do. Say the things you've always wanted to say.

This isn't an act or performance. You don't need to move a lot or bounce from position to position, although you can if that's what you're feeling. Just let your body move how it wants to. Follow the rhythms of the music. Grab a pillow if you want, and let it stand in for a woman. What do you want to say to her? Say it. "You feel so good. I fucking love you." Whatever it is, let yourself express it. You're completely alone, so there's no need to hold back. Explore the depths of your sexuality.

When you feel complete, let the image of your partner go. Give her a kiss and express your appreciation of the experience, then watch her fade away into the distance. Lie down and relax for a while to integrate the experience before returning to daily life.

Do this at least three times a week, giving yourself fully to your breath, sound, movement, and vocal expression. Before long, you'll see a big difference in how liberated you feel when you're in bed with an actual partner. It'll be easier to say the things you've always wanted to say. You're training your mind and body to be open and fully expressed.

EXERCISES TO CONNECT WITH A PARTNER

If you already have a partner and want to connect more deeply, there are so many ways to do that. In this section we'll cover a series of my favorites.

Examine Your Sexual Connection

At first, do this exercise privately. It's important for you to know yourself before you discuss the answers to the following questions with a partner. Before sharing them, create a context where it feels safe to give and receive feedback.

Ask yourself these questions:

- What's currently working well in your sexual connection with your partner?

- What do you feel is missing in your existing sexual connection with your partner?

- What else do you want to say to your partner about any aspect of your sex life, even if you feel that it's wrong? What do you deeply want to explore? What's holding you back from expressing yourself? Maybe there are things you did with a previous partner that you haven't yet felt comfortable mentioning to your current partner. Or you might be ashamed to ask for something, or afraid of hurting her feelings. Practice saying these things in the mirror, the shower, and during solo hikes before you bring them up with a partner. Think about how to express yourself with full conviction.

Your Perfect Sexual Day—And Hers

What have you always dreamed of exploring with a woman, even if you've never dared to express it? Take the time to write it down, in as much detail as possible. Put it in the form of a perfect sexual day or weekend.

Do you want her to wake you up by sucking your cock? Where will you go? What will you do? How would you like her to dress? What do you want to call her? Do you want to go find a secluded beach and fuck in the sand dunes? Or would you like to go to dinner at a fancy restaurant and have her return from the toilet and slip her soaking wet panties into your pocket? Let your imagination run wild here. In this scenario, don't focus on trying to please her. Just imagine what will turn you the fuck on.

This is absolutely for sharing. And it's only fair that she gets to do the same. Encourage her to do the exercise with you and agree on a time to share what you've both written.

Next, start acting out the list. Plan some time away and turn those sexual dreams into reality. You can do this by choosing one of you to go first—for example, by booking a weekend away and devoting one day to your fantasies and one to hers.

You can also create a joint perfect sexual day. This is where you talk about things you've always wanted to explore together and integrate them into one day. It doesn't have to be a combination of the things that are on your other lists, although it can be.

Need a little inspiration? Try out the four great sexual positions described at sexualquantumleap.com/resources.

The Five Senses Conversation

This is another great way to get to know what you like, what she likes, and what you'd like to explore together. Take a piece of paper and list the five senses: sight, hearing, smell, taste, and touch. Next to them, write down what turns you on in each of those categories.

Do you love to see your woman dressed in sexy lingerie, for example? What music do you like to hear in the bedroom? What words would you like her to whisper in your ear? Is there a favorite perfume she wears that drives you wild with desire? What foods turn you on? How do you like to touch and be touched?

Be as specific as possible and don't hold back. Create a list that you can use to fuel further adventures—we'll discuss these soon. Of course, encourage your partner to do this too.

INTENTIONAL SEX

Instead of leaping into bed after a busy workday, try using these exercises to drop into a sexual mood with your partner, connect deeply, and create a shared space.

Eye Contact

Stand at opposite ends of the room and make strong eye contact with your partner. Walk toward her slowly, with maximum presence, keeping the eye contact. Observe the sensations that arise as you get closer. You can also stop and match each other's breath. Play with the proximity, exploring how it feels to step forward and backward.

As you get closer, notice how much more intense the eye contact feels. You'll likely get fairly turned on purely from the physical closeness and eye contact. Feel like you're fucking her with your eyes. Hold the sexual tension for as long as you can both bear. Build the anticipation, with your faces inches apart. Sit in the sexual tension, breathe it in, and enjoy it. When the tension becomes so strong that you simply have to act on it, let desire guide you.

Breathe Together

First, set the mood with lighting and chill music. I like salt lamps and candles. Sit across from your partner in a comfortable seated position. Relax your face and take each other in visually. Really drop in and take the time to see each other. If you like, hold each other in a yab-yum or Yoda hug position, with her legs wrapped around your waist and a cushion under her butt.

Start by synchronizing your breath. Breathe deep belly breaths together for about five minutes, so you're in the same rhythm. Then, in the same position, do a round of Wim Hof breathing—thirty breaths. This will charge you both up and make you feel tingly.

When you're ready, lock lips with your partner and breathe into her mouth. She then breathes into your mouth, so you're sharing oxygen. It feels like you're one mouth, moving the air back and forth. Continue for as long as you can, then take a break. Alternate between Wim Hof breathing and sharing breath until you're both blissed out, for as many rounds as you want. At first, one round may be enough, but you can build up to more. You'll feel your whole body waking up and getting saturated with oxygen. It's deeply connecting and may feel like a natural psychedelic experience.

You'll start to feel high, deeply connected to your partner. At some point, you'll likely want to transition into kissing, making out, and having sex. Go with the flow. This exercise has led me to some of the most connected, transcendental sex I've experienced. It's almost cosmic and incredibly pleasurable.

Date Nights

You might think it's unsexy to plan sex in advance, but I think you'll be surprised. Set aside a night every week devoted purely to going on a date with your partner. In case you need some inspiration, refer back to your perfect sexual day, or explore an option from the Seven Nights of Sin below.

The rules of date night are that you can't talk about work or other personal worries. There's a time and a place for that kind of discussion. Instead, date nights are focused solely on the two of you, your connection, and your sex life. Talk about what turns you on and what you'd like to do. Discuss favorite sexual experiences you've shared, experiences you want to share together, and future sexual plans.

Take it in turns to lead the way. One week it's your turn to plan the experience, the next week it's hers, and the third it's a shared experience you create together. Yours-hers-ours in everything.

SEVEN NIGHTS OF SIN

In case you need some inspiration for ways to create a sexy mood, here come the Seven Nights of Sin. These are ideas you can steal to give yourself and a woman an amazing time. You don't need to do them all in one week—although it'll be a hell of a week if you do.

One: The Suited Gentleman

This is a chance to get dressed up and go out looking sharp. Pick out a classy suit, whether it's a three-piece or a tuxedo, and encourage the woman you're with to wear her most elegant gown.

Every woman has a dress that she loves, but it never seems to be the right time to wear it. Every woman has a pair of heels that she looks stunning in, but they're sitting in the back of her closet, unloved. How often do women get properly dressed up? On their wedding day and a few other special events throughout their lives. It's a rarity. This is that special occasion, when she can get dressed up to the nines and go out on the town with you.

Book a night in a quality hotel and make an event of it. Set the room up with candles, flowers, and strawberries; if you drink, get a nice bottle of champagne. There's no need to wait for a special occasion. Create one!

Start at a hip bar, end up at a fancy restaurant for dinner, and enjoy the feeling of everyone watching you because you look so good together. I used to do this in Melbourne, and it feels incredible, like owning the whole city.

To add an extra layer to the experience, get a vibrating egg that she inserts into her pussy, and have her wear it while you're out. You get to control the remote. Maybe you're at a posh restaurant and she's about to speak to the waiter when you turn on the vibrator and watch her reaction.

For extra points, get the hotel staff to fill the bath with rose petals and cue her favorite music while you're out, so that when you come back, she walks straight into an environment that turns her on even more.

Two: Fucking in Nature

This is a completely different vibe. Instead of feeling like the cream of society, get away from society completely. Go out into the middle of nowhere, where you're free to do exactly what you want, and let go.

I did this once at a secluded waterfall in Australia. She lay on the rocks by the waterfall while I fucked her like a savage, making her squirt, then put my fingers in her mouth, squeezing her tightly as the thunder boomed above us. It felt like we were ripping each other apart—a totally intoxicating experience. Both of us tapped into something deep and primal, screaming and yelling like untamed beasts. Then the rain came, along with thunder and lightning. We were drenched. It was a visceral experience.

Most of us spend the majority of our time dealing with the expectations of other people. It's such a relief to get naked, run free, and be wild. Nothing compares with bending a chick over an exposed tree root and fucking her while she screams with pleasure into the wild abyss. Some of my best dates have been taking women on dates in the wilderness with no one around but beautiful Mother Nature. Howl like the wild man you are and let loose your primal self. Encourage her to do the same. You can be Tarzan and she can be Jane, two savages in your element.

Three: Five Senses of Sin

This is a full-spectrum sensual experience, a night devoted to her pleasure. Remember we talked about the five senses earlier? You mapped out yours and she mapped out hers. This is where we're putting it to use. Your aim here is to stimulate her every sense.

Choose her favorite music—for added impact, play it through headphones so it's directly in her ears. Take her somewhere that excites her vision. What's she into? Art? Beautiful scenery? Whatever it is, find a way to feed that passion. Then think about the sense of touch. Does she like it when you rub an ice cube over her body? A sarong? Does she like to be scratched?

Try blindfolding her to increase the response from her other senses. It takes about twenty minutes of wearing a blindfold for all her other senses to heighten. Give her something she loves to taste, such as a piece of exquisite chocolate. Ideally, plan a whole sequence of experiences for her and lead her through them one by one.

Of course, she'll want to reciprocate and do the same for you, too, which is why I got you to understand what triggers your five senses.

Four: Sensual Massage

Women love a guy who knows how to give a great massage. I highly recommend taking a massage course to learn some basic techniques. Tell women that you're looking for someone to practice your massage skills on, and you'll have no shortage of volunteers.

That said, don't feel like you need to do some training before you touch a woman. There's no need to have perfect technique. If all you do is apply some coconut or sesame oil and run your hands over her body, that'll still feel really good for her.

Make sure you set the right mood for this. Play soft music and light some candles, so she gets into a relaxed frame of mind. To prepare for the massage, you may want to put down some towels so you don't get oil on your bedsheets. Start with your hands on her lower back and invite her to take some deep breaths so she can drop into her body.

When you get the oil out, always warm it up with your hands. Don't just pour it onto her body cold. This is a sensual massage, so take it slow. Don't just go straight for her pussy. If she's comfortable letting you massage her body, sex is on the cards. Don't rush it and ruin the moment.

For an even more amazing experience, try body slides. Slather each other in high-quality coconut or sesame oil and slide all over her body. Sesame oil is warming, whereas coconut oil has a cooling feel.

You can take it to the next level by running a hot bath for her afterward and filling it with flowers and bubble bath. Alternatively, lead her to the bedroom, ask her to lie down and close her eyes, and drop flowers on her body. These kinds of touches make a woman feel seriously special.

Once you're in the zone, you may want to give her a pussy massage. This is a famous—perhaps infamous—way to send a woman into ecstasy. The pussy massage alone is probably the easiest and most effective way to give a woman the most insane sexual experience of her life and likely send her into multiorgasmic bliss. You'll find our explanatory video at sexualquantumleap.com/resources.

Five: Live Out a Fantasy

Number five on the Seven Nights of Sin is excellent practice for knowing and asking for what you want. It's also a way to let your darker fantasies surface. Like the perfect sexual day or weekend, this is an opportunity to connect both with your desires and hers. One night is yours, the next hers, and the third is collaborative.

When it's your turn, give your girl highly specific instructions about what you'd like her to do. For example, tell her what makeup and lingerie to wear, right down to the color of her nails and how you want her to style her hair, then instruct her to put on a trench coat and come to your house.

Another option: book a hotel for the night, give her the key, and let her know exactly how and when you want her to wait for you. For example: "I want you to wait for me facedown on the bed, with your ass in the air, wearing the matching set of underwear I gave you for your birthday."

The possibilities here are endless. The only limit is your imagination. If you have a role-play fantasy, try it out. Ask her to dress as Little Red Riding Hood while you play the big bad wolf or become a teacher while she plays the sexy student. Maybe you want to be the doctor who gives his patient a very thorough examination, or she likes the idea of being an unusually attentive nurse. Request what you want and let her tell you whether she's comfortable with it.

Six: Master Chef

Sexuality is about so much more than just sex. It's about anticipation and building up eroticism. Food and sex are deeply interlinked, so it makes sense that great food and great sex combine perfectly. I tested out this idea with a partner. We had a night where we ate pizza together and fucked. It was pretty good. Then, another night, we made a menu out of foods that are known as aphrodisiacs and ate those together, to see the difference. It was like night and day.

You can have some fun with this by cooking together, perhaps naked except for your aprons. Take pride in what you create and make it as high quality as possible. Seafood is a good choice for an aphrodisiac. Try oysters to start, followed by a prawn salad with lots of leafy greens. If you drink alcohol, pair it with a nice white wine. And make it playful, by feeding each other to tantalize your senses, for example.

For dessert, try strawberries coated in dark chocolate. Chocolate is a natural aphrodisiac; the darker the chocolate, the more powerful the effect. Rub the strawberries on each other's lips before feeding them to each other. It's hot as hell. You can even get a block of chocolate and lie on top of her until your body heat melts the chocolate, then lick it off each other.

Seven: On the Seventh Day...

There are actually only six nights of sin. If you've worked your way through all of those, you deserve a rest. Even God rested on the seventh day; you can, too.

ALWAYS BE A STUDENT

As I've said previously, there's nothing special about me. I'm not smarter than you. I've learned the ideas in this chapter from mentors, tried them myself, shared them with clients, and now written about them for you.

I see myself as a sexual detective, constantly exploring what creates a great experience. I'm willing to ask the questions most guys don't and continually untangle my sexuality, along with the sexuality of the guys I work with and the women I meet.

I always have at least one sexuality mentor in my life. I find the best in the world at whatever I want to learn more about, pay them what they want, apply whatever they teach me, then teach it to you. I made a choice to work exceptionally hard on this part of myself and I'm still learning. Sexuality is such a deep rabbit hole, and I still feel like a virgin every day. If someone tells you they know everything there is to know about sexuality, don't believe them. There's always more to know.

At the same time, no one knows your sexuality better than you. The exercises in this chapter are inroads to discovering yourself and your partners sexually. You might be terrified of trying some of these at first, but if you do them, they will bring you sexual confidence and charisma you've never known before.

You might feel locked up, in your head and/or your body. In time, these exercises will change that. You can let go of the need to be someone you're not and come to appreciate who you are sexually. Keep chipping away. This stuff works. I've taken you to water, motherfucker. Now it is time to drink.

LUSTY'S STORY: PART II

Today, Lusty regularly has experiences he would never have believed were possible. After we started working together, he began going to sex parties and exploring all kinds of crazy shit in the bedroom. Before long, he was *running* sex parties with me. He had women lining up to play with him, more than he could handle.

When COVID-19 hit, he moved back home with his parents. In the past, this would have been a cue for him to sink back into sexual repression. Instead, he found a way to keep exploring and having incredible experiences.

He got to enjoy his first threesome, with one chick on her knees sucking him off while the other one sat on his shoulders, wrapping her legs around him as he ate her pussy. When his dad came home earlier than expected, he was forced to run into his room and lock the door. His parents wondered what was going on and he told them the girls were just friends, but they suspected there was more to it.

The list of Lusty's lustful experiences is far longer than I can cover in this book but suffice to say that he can make any woman he wants squirt. Women call him up all the time because they want the pleasure he can give them.

One night, he called me because he had a girl at his house. He was exhausted and she was still horny, so he brought her over to me—I live about twenty minutes from him—and tapped me in. Another time, he brought a girl from a nightclub into my hotel room, where me, Black Mamba, and another chick turned it into a group thing. On multiple occasions, Lusty has brought women to me because he needed a break.

The reason I'm sharing these examples is not to boast. It's to show you what's possible. When I met him, Lusty was short, fat, and chronically lacking in confidence. He never would have believed that he could have the kind of experiences I'm describing. Now, he has women wondering where they'll ever find another man like him. He has also overcome a chronic porn addiction and a problem with premature ejaculation, enhancing his business success in the process.

Incidentally, he hasn't confined himself to short-term experiences. He has also had two longer-term partners since we met. Your sexual ambitions may or may not match Lusty's. Perhaps you're looking for one great partner for life. Whatever you want, however, realize that if he can live out so many of his wildest sexual fantasies, you can too.

7

INSIDE AND OUTSIDE THE BEDROOM

Billy thought he was a real bad boy.

We met through a mutual friend—a dating coach—in Bali. I could see that, behind the mask he sometimes put on, he was a great, down-to-earth guy. He was fun, charismatic, and he'd had a lot of sexual experiences in his life, but something was missing. Because I'm a sex coach, we inevitably got talking about his sex life.

He told me that he already had great sex, but he was open-minded about possible improvements. Although he wasn't sure exactly *what* he could do better, he felt that there was another level available to him. Billy was heavily into personal development and he was constantly looking for ways to level up.

The more he told me, the clearer it became that he was holding back from asking for what he wanted. He often got drunk or high before he had sex, which allowed him to relax but detracted from his presence. He thought that, as a man, it was his responsibility to give the women he fucked a great experience. Although his assertiveness allowed women to relax, he was struggling for deep connection. He didn't know how to feel deeply, relax, or allow women to fully relax with him.

Billy didn't know what he didn't know. He wasn't seeing that the way he fucked in the bedroom was the way he fucked life. Initially, he was skeptical about working with me. He wasn't sure what I could show him that he wasn't already seeing. That changed after he attended a free event I ran. He applied some of the ideas I discussed and, a couple nights later, went out and ended up going home with a beautiful Russian chick.

He took me out for dinner to tell me about it. "Dude," he told me, "I went to this chick's house and fucked. It was easily the best sexual experience of my life. She was going crazy. Afterward, as we were lying in bed catching our breath, she turned to me and said, 'Are you a sex coach?' I was looking for the hidden cameras because I thought you'd set me up!"

After that, he decided to go all in on my teachings.

From that point, Billy's sex life changed beyond recognition. A couple of weeks later, he met a new woman who became his girlfriend for a while. By this time, we were living together, so I had tangible evidence of her enjoyment. The whole house used to shake when they fucked.

Billy told me he'd never had a sexual experience like that, and neither had she. The difference? Instead of locking up his emotions, he started expressing himself in the bedroom. He gave his voice free rein. That simple shift invited a whole new level of connection.

Billy knew lots of techniques. He knew how to give women orgasms. But he had been shutting himself down, and women didn't feel safe to completely express themselves with him. After we worked together, he gave himself permission to say the things he'd always wanted to say. The difference was like night and day.

BRINGING IT ALL TOGETHER

By now you know this isn't a relationship book, but I want to leave you with an understanding of the way your sexual connections with women interact with your connections outside the bedroom.

It's great to be the best she ever had sexually, but if you want her to love you, stay with you, and insist on seeing you again, you'll need to be a man she respects and admires outside the bedroom, too. In this chapter, we're going to lay out The Sexual Quantum Leap Pyramid (we'll call it The SQL Pyramid from now on) and The Love Code. The SQL Pyramid will help you to understand exactly where you are as a man, and where there are gaps in your development. The Love Code will bring the information in The SQL Pyramid into context, giving you another way to relate to it and apply it in your daily life.

No doubt you'll recognize some of what we talk about in this chapter. This chapter is a cross between a refresher course and a high-level summary. The value of The SQL Pyramid and The Love Code is that they give you frameworks for everything we've discussed throughout the book. If you ever want to put anything you've read here in context, refer to The SQL Pyramid and The Love Code, and it will instantly make sense.

That doesn't mean you *have* to use these concepts to find a long-term partner. If you want a casual lover, you can still blow her mind in bed. But if you *want* a long-term partner, you need to understand other aspects of female psychology. In this chapter, we'll break down all those distinctions so you can send the right signals to the right women.

If you've skipped over the rest of the book to get to this section, I recommend going back and reading the previous chapters. Everything laid out here will make a lot more sense if you already understand the background behind it.

THE SEXUAL QUANTUM LEAP PYRAMID

This really is some of the most profound material I know. It tracks the stages of a man's development. Use it well and you will be in a great position to consistently be the best she ever had, inside and outside the bedroom. More than that. You'll be able to consistently enjoy experiences that are the best *you* ever had.

When you make use of the insights in The SQL Pyramid and The Love Code, women will fall head over heels in love with you. With great power comes great responsibility, so make sure you act in the best interests of the women you meet.

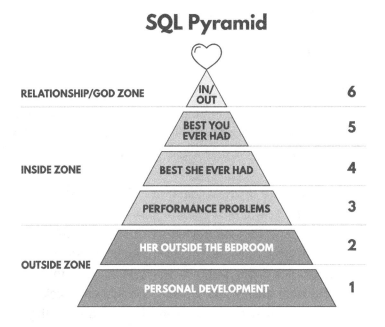

The SQL Pyramid consists of three zones: Outside the Bedroom, Inside the Bedroom, and the God/Relationship Zone. These three zones break down into six stages. From bottom to top, these are:

- **Stage 1:** Personal Development

- **Stage 2:** Her Outside the Bedroom

- **Stage 3:** Performance Problems

- **Stage 4:** Best She Ever Had

- **Stage 5:** Best You Ever Had

- **Stage 6:** In/Out

Although there is a progression up the pyramid, it's not linear. You may be really strong in Stage 4, but still have some work to do in Stage 1. Laid out like this, you can see where you're killing it and where you still have work to do.

Stage 1 and 2 are grouped together in Zone 1: the Outside Zone. Stages 3, 4, and 5 come under the umbrella of the Inside Zone, and Stage 6 stands alone in the Relationship/ God Zone. If this all sounds a bit confusing, don't worry. We're going to break it down, stage by stage, in this chapter. We'll talk about what each stage entails, how you can track your progress through each stage, and—best of all—what you will hear yourself and women saying in each stage. This isn't just hypothetical. You'll hear and use these exact phrases, or variations on them, as you move through The SQL Pyramid. They are a great benchmark of your progress.

Stage 1: Personal Development

It's essential that you work on your personal development and continually become a better man. Personally, I've spent hundreds of thousands of dollars on this area of my life and never regretted the investment.

We've talked a lot about what makes a man, such as self-respect, honesty, and the ability to show up. A consistent commitment to improving yourself is just as important. However much money you have in the bank, however many women you've been with, what ultimately defines you is your character.

You probably wouldn't have picked up this book without a strong interest in personal development. You know how important it is. That's why it forms the foundation of The SQL Pyramid.

Mastering Stage 1

As you begin to knock it out of the park in Stage 1, you'll find that you're consistently on purpose. You'll feel like everything you spend your time on contributes to a bigger mission. You'll be living an inspired life, showing up with integrity. Your thoughts, words, and actions will be aligned.

Your health, wealth, and relationships will be on point, and you'll effortlessly exhibit many of the character traits we've already described in these pages. For example, you'll be a nice guy with boundaries and a benevolent leader, building up the people around you and making them better. You'll be unafraid of expressing what you want. You'll be connected with an infectious sense of aliveness. Yet, you'll also be humble, willing to adopt a beginner's mindset and acknowledge what you don't know.

What You Will Say and Hear in Stage 1

You will say:

- "I feel inspired, on purpose, and on my mission."

- "I feel like my life has meaning and a strong direction."

- "I know what I want and where I'm going."

- "I'm surrounded by people who love, support, and respect me."

- "I feel alive and aligned with who I am."

She will say:

- "You are a genius."

- "You are such an incredible man."

- "I am inspired by you."

Stage 2: Her Outside the Bedroom

Stage 2 is about knowing your woman outside the bedroom. It's about understanding the totality of who she is, not just how to please her sexually.

Just as there's so much more to you than your sexuality, there's much more to her, too. It's amazing to be the best she ever had, but if you really want to inspire her heart and mind, you'll need to know who she is as a person, on every level.

This will have an impact on how open she is to you inside the bedroom, too. When she trusts you to know her deeply and authentically outside the bedroom, she'll be willing to give herself to you deeply on a sexual level.

Mastering Stage 2

How do you truly get to know a woman? Ask her questions. Get curious about her wants, needs, fears, and desires. What does she think about first thing in the morning and last thing at night?

Get a sense of her childhood. What was it like to be her as a child? Did she find it easy? Hard? What did she like about her upbringing? What didn't she like? What relationships are most important to her? Who is she closest to? Family? Friends? Understand what makes those connections special.

What is important to her? What are her goals, values, and mission? Don't rely purely on what she says. Observe her behavior. What does she prioritize? You can learn so much about someone from seeing what inspires them, what lights them up, and what moves them. What does she love to do? Why? For something to be her favorite thing, there must be a powerful reason. It's an amazing turn-on for a man to be with a woman who's inspired by her life.

As you get to know her more deeply, delve into the key milestones of her life, and her biggest peaks and valleys. What are the moments that have shaped her? In what way? Don't be afraid to take an interest in the darker times. Most of the time, we humans avoid the shittier parts of life, but they shape us in essential ways. You can't know a woman without knowing about her dark times.

How does she imagine her future? What are her aspirations? Keep asking why and digging in deeper to truly understand her. Invite her to paint a picture for you.

What You Will Hear in Stage 2

She will say:

- "You know me better than any other man."

- "You know me even better than my girlfriends and family."

- "I've never shared this with anyone before."

- "You make me feel so safe and comfortable."

- "I feel like I can tell you anything."

- "I feel like you really understand me."

- "I feel like I've known you my whole life."

- "It's like you know me better than I know myself."

- "You just get me."

Stage 3: Performance Problems

Now we're moving inside the bedroom. Not every guy has performance issues. If you don't struggle with PE, ED, or delayed ejaculation, that's great. For guys who do, however, handling this stuff is fundamental to being the best she ever had, and to having the best experiences of their lives.

A lot of guys wonder why we don't put this right at the bottom of The SQL Pyramid. The reason is that you can be a god in the bedroom, but if you don't have the fundamentals sorted, women won't stick around for the long-term. Work on who you are as a man, and on deeply knowing the woman in front of you, and you'll have a strong bond. If you don't do that, you will always rely on your performance to keep women around, which is a lot of pressure.

This stage also covers the pressure that comes with focusing on performance, not presence.

Mastering Stage 3

By now, you're probably familiar with performance issues. Premature ejaculation means you cum too quickly, before sex starts or within a few pumps. Erectile dysfunction means you can't get it up or keep it up. Delayed ejaculation means you can't cum in the bedroom. Maybe you get nervous or stuck in your head and you can't relax enough to reach an orgasm.

As we discussed in the previous chapter, performance issues can have mental, emotional, and physical causes. Sometimes more than one. There are different remedies depending on the source of the problem, but whatever it is, you're not fucked up, and you're not broken. There are natural solutions. Your refractory period will naturally increase with age, but it shouldn't feel like you're struggling to get hard.

When you're mastering this stage, you should feel relaxed and present in sexual situations. Instead of being anxious and stuck in your head, you'll be confident that you can get and stay hard when you want to, without reaching orgasm before you and your partner are ready. You'll be at ease, able to focus on being the best she ever had—and the best you ever had. In other words, you'll be able to get it up and keep it up as long as you want, last as long as you want, and cum whenever you want, because you are relaxed and in control.

What You Will Say and Think in Stage 3

You will say and think:

- "I can last as long as I want."

- "I have rock-hard erections."

- "I can control when I cum."

- "I can get it up and keep it up when I fuck."

- "I have stronger erections."

- "I no longer feel pressure to perform."

- "I feel relaxed and enjoy the sexual experience."

- "I feel present in the bedroom."

- "I can reload quicker and go all night."

Stage 4: Best She Ever Had

By now, you should be familiar with the content in this stage. Throughout the book, we've discussed numerous aspects of being the best she ever had. We've talked about how every woman is different, and every pussy is different. We've covered the Yours-Hers-Ours model of sexuality. It begins with you, extends to her, and culminates in cocreation.

We've discussed how women love to feel desired, and how much a woman needs to know that you crave her, and how you can please a woman using your tongue, your fingers, and your cock. Chapter Six, Practical Ways to Boost Your Sex Life, is packed with ideas you can use to be the best she ever had, and the links scattered throughout the book will take you to content you can apply straightaway. There are a million ways to be the best she ever had.

Mastering Stage 4

Mastery in this stage consists of what you were probably expecting when you picked up this book—consistently giving women the best sexual experiences of their lives. When you're flowing in this stage, you'll be a dominant man with deep sexual confidence. You'll be a genius at going slow and creating sexual tension. You'll be a foreplay magician who can turn her on so much she's begging you to fuck her. And when you *do* fuck her, you'll be able to make her cum multiple times.

You'll know how to use your tongue, fingers, and toys to give her incredible pleasure, not just your cock. You'll be skilled at turning her on with messages, so she's gagging to fuck you before you even get together.

When it comes to communication and negotiation, you'll be a star. You'll get to know the women you have sex with intimately, asking the hard questions and saying the hard things, so you can understand what they want and how they want it. How do they like to be touched, teased, and fucked? You'll dive into and understand her sexuality on a profound level, so you have a comprehensive picture of the woman in front of you, including her wildest fantasies and kinks.

Ultimately, you'll know her sexually better than she knows herself, and be able to give women multiple orgasms every time and know that you truly are the best she's ever had.

What You Will Hear in Stage 4

She will say:

- "You're the best I ever had."

- "I've never had that many orgasms before."

- "Wow, what the fuck was that? You're seriously a sex god."

- "When's round two?"

- "You've ruined me for other men."

- "My girlfriends are going to be so jealous when I tell them."

- "I can't even remember the last time a man fucked me like that. I'm not going to be able to walk properly for the next few days."

- "Fuck, I screamed so loud your neighbors are going to hate me."

- "I'm going to be thinking about that experience for the rest of my life."

- "I've never felt this way with any other man."

Stage 5: Best You Ever Had

A lot of men, especially high-performing men, neglect this stage. They get so focused on giving a woman a great experience that they forget to stop and think about their own experience. This is why it's so important to integrate the material in Chapter Four, Knowing and Asking for What You Want.

It's easy to be the best she ever had. The bar's so low. Most guys just put it in, thrust away for a few minutes, and cum. If you can do even a tenth of what we teach at SQL, you'll be miles ahead of the game. Being the best you ever had is some next-level shit.

Until you truly understand what turns you on, how can you communicate it to a woman? If you don't know what you like, and you spend all your time performing for a woman, you'll gradually become resentful, wondering when you will get your needs met. You may not even be able to fully articulate why you feel the way you do, but it will poison your connections with women.

That's why this stage is so important. It's the most neglected, and absolutely key to creating and sharing experiences that will not only be the best she ever had, but also the best *you* ever had. Paradoxically, when sex is the best you ever had, you'll feel so relaxed and comfortable that you'll easily be the best she ever had. A woman wants nothing more than to see you let go, flow, and allow pleasure to take over your body.

Mastering Stage 5

To play in this stage, you'll need to understand how you want to be touched, teased, and fucked. What turns you on? What are your fantasies? What really gets you going? What are your wants, needs, and curiosities? What really scratches that itch?

When there's something you want, do you go for it? Do you know how to ask? Have you completed the exercises in this book, such as your perfect sexual day? Are you in touch with your fantasies and kinks? What do you want to explore sexually? What do you want her to say and do to you?

Whatever your desires are, it's so important that you know them, that you can express them, and that you can negotiate for them. Your unapologetic approval of your own sexuality will pave the way for her to wholeheartedly approve of and connect with you sexually. You may not even have a lot of crazy kinks and fantasies. If not, that's okay. What's important is that you know what you like—and, if you're not sure, that you take the time to find out.

What You Will Say and Think in Stage 5

You will say and think:

- "That was the best sexual experience of my life."

- "That was the best orgasm I've ever had."

- "That was the most meaningful sex I've ever had."

- "I gave myself permission to explore my sexuality."

- "I'm glad I tried that."

- "I've never experienced that much pleasure."

- "I never thought I'd feel this way."

- "I felt so free, that was fucking amazing."

- "That was the biggest load I have ever shot."

- "I've never had a woman look at me like that before."

Stage 6: Relationship/God Zone

At the top of The SQL Pyramid is Stage 6. Stage 6 is the space you'll inhabit more and more consistently as you work on all aspects of The SQL Pyramid. It's an integration of everything that's come before, so you will only get to this place when you're ready to take an honest, unflinching look at the places you're falling short, and take action to address them.

I call it the Relationship/God Zone because, when you're living in this place, you'll be able to attract incredible women and continuously deepen your connections with them. If you decide to select one woman and build something amazing together, you'll have no difficulty keeping her around. She'll see you as relationship material because of who you are outside the bedroom, and a sex god because of who you are inside the bedroom.

Mastering Stage 6

The only thing you don't do with your best friend is have sex. When you reach Stage 6, you'll be able to form connections with women that have all the trust and empathy of a best friendship, plus all the heat and passion of an incredible sexual connection.

You'll both be living inspired, purposeful lives. You'll have any performance issues handled. The sex will be the best she ever had and the best you ever had. You'll feel met by her, inside and outside the bedroom. You'll build each other up and make each other better, day after day. With a little effort—using the exercises in this book—you'll be able to sustain the honeymoon phase for life, sharing peaks of emotional and sexual connection and becoming an ever more powerful team.

What You Will Say and Hear in Stage 6

You and she will say:

- "You're amazing, inside and outside the bedroom."

- "You know every aspect of me."

- "I've never met someone like you before."

- "Where have you been my whole life?"

- "I love you so much."

- "Thank you for knowing and accepting every part of me."

- "You know exactly how to satisfy all my needs."

- "You're my man."

- "You're the man I want to spend the rest of my life with."

- "I want to start a family and grow old with you."

Summarizing The SQL Pyramid

I hope you've been nodding along as you read through this chapter. The reason I put it together is so that you can use it to pinpoint where you're on the right track and where you need to put in some work.

Every aspect of your sexual relationships can be plotted on The SQL Pyramid, and everything in this book fits in there. It unfolds endlessly, constantly yielding new insights, and you'll never reach the end. There's always more to do, more to learn, and deeper insights to uncover at each stage. For a more in-depth look into The SQL Pyramid, click on the link at sexualquantumleap.com/resources.

THE LOVE CODE

There's a lot of crossover between the Sexual Quantum Leap Pyramid and The Love Code. The Love Code breaks the content in The SQL Pyramid into two separate triangles: Inside the Bedroom and Outside the Bedroom.

Each one of those triangles consists of three parts: Yours, Hers, and Ours. This is because, as we've discussed, all these aspects are essential. You need to know yourself, know

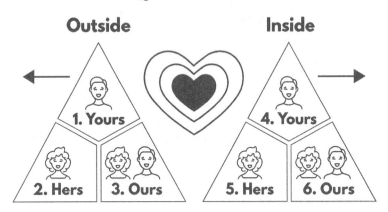

her, and together you can build a connection that is a unique combination of the two of you.

The triangle shape is a reminder that, if one of these aspects is missing, the whole thing falls apart. The pieces slot together to become something bigger and more powerful as a whole than they are on their own. The more that you focus on the qualities defined by each triangle, the bigger the heart in the middle grows—and the more in love you will both feel.

Outside the Bedroom

Outside the bedroom, how well do you know yourself? This connects with Stage 1 of The SQL Pyramid. Are you developing yourself? Are you on purpose? Do you feel inspired by the life you're living, every day? Does she respect you?

To love you, a woman needs to respect your character, your integrity, and your mission. If your goal is to meet one great woman and spend the rest of your life with her, great sex won't be enough. You'll need to be someone she admires in every aspect of your life.

How well do you know her? This is Stage 2 of The SQL Pyramid. What lights her up? Is she living a life that consistently connects her with her passions? Unless you truly know what brings her joy, how will you form a healthy, loving relationship?

Encourage her to show you who she truly is. When she does, accept and celebrate her. I spoke to a guy recently who was bummed because he felt that his partner didn't appreciate him. I asked him whether he ever appreciated *her*. When he realized that he didn't, he made an effort to show his partner more appreciation. Before long, he was receiving more appreciation from her.

When you come together in relationship, that connects to Stage 6. If you're both living your best life, you know all aspects of each other outside the bedroom, and you're constantly diving deeper and deeper into intimate discovery, you're living the relationship dream.

Inside the Bedroom

We've already talked at length about how sexuality starts with you, and how important it is that you know yourself sexually. Do you know what you like, and are you sharing it with your partner? Are you negotiating for the things you want to try? Do you fully accept yourself sexually?

As you can see, this connects with Stage 5, the most neglected stage of The SQL Pyramid. When you see it as a piece of The Love Code, hopefully you understand that it's not optional. Without doing the work to examine, explore, and express your sexuality, you'll never complete the puzzle.

Everything starts with knowing yourself. Sexually speaking, that means understanding what you like and what you want. It means unapologetically owning those truths, even if you think they're weird. It means having the courage to open up and be vulnerable with women you like.

Her sexuality connects with Stage 4 on The SQL Pyramid. Are you leading her with love? Are you taking the time to understand her sexually? To create date nights that take you both to new places sexually? Are you open to hearing what she has to tell you about the things she'd like to do?

Enjoy and appreciate her sexuality, and her willingness to share it with you. When you're with a woman, give her full permission to express herself sexually. Show her, with your words and your actions, that you fully welcome all aspects of her sexuality.

Of course, the final piece of the puzzle is how you come together (no pun intended). How does the combination of your sexual energy and hers look and feel? When you collaborate on a date night, how does it take you to unexpected heights that neither of you could have reached alone? This connects to Stage 6 of The SQL Pyramid, representing the pinnacle of your shared sexual experiences.

USING THE LOVE CODE

The Love Code shows you what to focus on when you want to build a sexual connection, and what to focus on when you want to build a relationship.

If you concentrate on what happens outside the bedroom, you'll be an amazing man, you'll meet amazing women, and you'll be able to build deep and fulfilling friendships. This is not to say you'll be stuck in the friend zone. There may be women in your life who you want to nurture deep friendships with, but don't feel drawn to sexually. If so, great. Just focus on Yours-Hers-Ours outside the bedroom.

Alternatively, there may be times when you want to connect with a woman on a purely sexual level. Okay, your main focus will be on the Inside the Bedroom triangle. Understanding and expressing your sexuality, encouraging her to do the same, and combining those to create an incredible sexual experience.

When you combine both of these aspects, you're on track to build an incredible relationship. They will naturally feed off each other, enhancing your connection. When your presence outside the bedroom complements the sexual experiences you're sharing inside the bedroom, it's like rocket fuel. And just like rocket fuel, you need to be careful with it.

When you've got The Love Code going for you, it's game over. Don't turn it all on unless you're serious about the woman you're with. Otherwise, you may break a few hearts. Sometimes people misconstrue these ideas as manipulative. That's not my intention at all. They're a road map for creating amazing experiences with women. But they should always be used ethically.

With great power there must also come great responsibility. Don't mislead women. If all you want is a beautiful fuck buddy relationship, that's totally cool. Represent yourself honestly. On the other hand, if you're looking for a path into something deeper and more meaningful, The Love Code shows you how to get there.

BILLY'S STORY: PART II

Billy has put his newfound sex god status to good use. He's met a woman with whom he has an amazing, deep, beautiful connection. She keeps him accountable for being the best possible man. They vibe completely, inside and outside the bedroom. He's into health and wellness and she's a yoga teacher and holistic therapist, so they're perfectly compatible.

It's so great that I feel slightly jealous. There's so much love and reverence between them. I can see it in the way they kiss. They're not perfect. Like any relationship, they work on stuff. But they're pretty damn good. They're doing the work, and the more they dive into their relationship, the better it gets for them.

They also have a great story about how they met. The first time they saw each other was at a club in Bali. They hung out and chatted a bit without taking it anywhere. The next time Billy saw her she was at a bar. He decided it was time to be a bit bolder, so he walked right up to her and said, "Hey, I think you're sexy. We should get to know each other better."

She looked at him and said, "Huh?" It turns out she's an identical twin. Billy walked up to the wrong twin and made a move. Out of the corner of his eye, Billy saw another girl who looked exactly like the one he was talking to, and it started to dawn on him what was happening. "I think you're looking for my sister," said the twin. "I think you're right," Billy responded. Fortunately, it wasn't the first case of mistaken identity they'd known. They all laughed about it later.

The major difference for Billy is his capacity to connect emotionally. It was one thing to be good in bed, but now he feels as though his entire life has another dimension. He feels true intimacy. He's in a relationship with a woman who cares deeply about him, and who he cares about deeply. They plan to get married and one day have kids together.

8

LEAVE HER BETTER
AND WETTER

When I met Ryko, he thought he'd never love again.

He met his first girlfriend when he was fourteen. At that age, she was the love of his life. Tragically, she died suddenly when she was sixteen, an event that scarred Ryko for decades.

We bumped into each other at a hippie festival in Australia, when he was forty-five. I was there with Black Mamba. We were there to have fun and crazy sexual experiences. Ryko hung out with us a bit. He was a nice guy with a good heart and a gentle soul, but nervous and shy.

Following the death of his childhood sweetheart, Ryko patched himself up as best he could. He got married and had a kid, even though deep down he knew there was something missing. The marriage broke down. When we met, he was trying to find himself. The more time he spent with us, the more he realized what he was missing out on.

One night, Black Mamba, Butterfly Heart, another friend, and I were hanging out with several chicks. There were three of us in a giant cuddle puddle with about ten chicks. Eventually, all but two of them left, and it was on.

At one point, Black Mamba and Butterfly Heart were fucking one of the chicks each, while I lay between them stroking the women. I remember having sex with one of them, a dread-locked mostly-lesbian, who started making an incredible amount of noise. There were people walking down the path close by who could hear everything. Laughingly, I commented that she was making a lot of noise. She yelled back, "I don't give a fuck!"

Ryko heard and saw all of this, along with six or eight of our friends in the campsite, and it awakened something in him. He wanted to join in, but he didn't have the confidence. He longed for the love he hadn't felt since he was a teenager, but he also loved the idea of having some crazy fun with some amazing women. He lacked presence and, most of the time, women didn't give him the time of day. They didn't respect him.

Fast forward three or four months, and we connected for a chat. He confessed that he wanted sexual experiences like the ones he'd witnessed at the festival. We went out for dinner and talked it through, and he decided to come to a retreat. At the time, I didn't know the full story of his first love, nor under-stand how much it had shut him down.

At the retreat, Ryko opened up to me about the experience. He admitted that he'd never fully processed it and that, even three decades later, it still had an impact on his ability to open up to women. Outwardly, he'd moved on with his life. Inwardly, he was still the same wounded teenager he had been since his girlfriend passed away.

BE A POSITIVE INFLUENCE

We're coming to the end of the book. It's time to talk about being a positive influence in a woman's life. It doesn't matter whether you see her for one night, for five years, or for a lifetime. Leave her life better for having known you.

Whatever the container, how can you create an experience you'll both cherish? Can you allow yourself to open up and explore a real, deep connection? Can you lead with benevolence and invite a woman to show you her true self? Can you build her up so that she feels better about herself and her sexuality for knowing you?

If you can do all the above, and take a genuine interest in her sexuality, you'll both thrive on the connection you build together. She'll be excited to see you again. Whether you spend a lifetime together or go your separate ways the next morning, you'll be improved by the experience, and so will she.

It's important to admit here that I'm no angel. I've fucked up many times and there are plenty of women in the world who would say that I haven't left them better and wetter. I haven't always stood up to be counted on as a man. I've cheated and lied and done stupid things.

I still feel bad about some of the things I've done, but I can't change the past. All I can do is forgive myself for past mistakes, learn, and do better in the future.

SEXUAL TRUST

We've already talked in detail about ways you can encourage a woman to relax. Back tickles, face touching, slow caresses, massage. All of these can build sexual trust. Diversity of touch is important. Scratches, squeezes, hugs, caresses—all are ways to create connection without signaling sexual urgency.

The fundamental principle is that you're not trying to force anything. When you take your time and enjoy each moment, you'll allow a woman to do the same. She won't feel like you're trying to get something from her.

If she comes to your place, offer her a drink and give her a tour. Be curious about who she is, and not just sexually. See her as a unique human being. Encourage her to express herself by asking questions and being willing to share yourself vulnerable.

Sometimes you might find that the energy between you doesn't lead to sex. Can you be okay with that, and simply enjoy whatever you share? If you can, she'll think of you as a cool guy who she can trust, and she'll likely want to see you again.

Building sexual trust/tension doesn't mean coming off as asexual—the nice guy who doesn't have the courage to ask for what he wants. You still have boundaries and you're connected with your sexuality. You're not afraid of intensity or passion. But you know how to handle yourself sexually and inject sexual tension into a connection with a woman.

If you're scared you're stuck in the dreaded friend zone, look objectively at the situation. Are you hanging out alone together with a glass of wine? Is she comfortable with you? How does she react when you move closer to her, make a sexually suggestive comment about her appearance, hold strong eye contact, or pick her up physically as you hug her? A woman who comes to your house in a dating context is likely ready to be seduced. It's on you to lead the way and make it smooth and seamless.

The friend zone is a place for men who are scared of expressing themselves sexually and try to win a woman's affection in underhanded ways. Like we said, nice guys who pretend they're not interested in women sexually are lying to themselves. Women will pick up on their ulterior motives and get turned off. Now that you've read this book, that's never going to be you, right?

SAFETY PRECAUTIONS

We've talked about the importance of safe words and consent. It would be wrong of me to end this book without emphasizing that one more time. Consent is absolutely paramount. Don't ever try to force a woman to do anything she's uncomfortable with. If she pulls away, get curious and ask what's happening. Dial it back so that she knows you're not going to do anything that might hurt her. I trust that you know the difference between a woman who's saying no and a woman who's teasing you playfully.

If she's looking at you devilishly, unzipping your pants, and saying, "We shouldn't be doing this," you can be pretty sure that she wants to. If she's backing away, looking genuinely concerned, and saying "stop," she doesn't.

Many women love to create plausible deniability. A woman may tell you that she "hardly ever does this" or that you "bring out the bad girl" in her, all while messaging you at 11:00 p.m. saying she is bored. When you invite her over to drink wine on your balcony, she knows what's happening, but she can tell herself that it's an innocent chat, so she doesn't feel like a slut. I can't count the number of times I've invited a woman over for wine, only for her to bring condoms and wear her sexiest lingerie. Women aren't stupid. They know what's happening. They just don't want to be explicit about it. I've even questioned women on this after we've had sex, and—after the fact—they usually admit that of course they were coming over to fuck.

The next day, she can report back to her friends that it "just happened!" It's a little sad that women feel so scared of judgment that they need to put up these defenses, but it's worth understanding them for what they are. As an aside, you can playfully turn this attitude around, by telling women you're shy and they're being naughty by turning you on, as a way to tease them and amp up the sexual tension. This will only work if you're sexually confident, not if you're genuinely shy and nervous.

When things start to heat up, don't be afraid to have an honest conversation. Let's say you're kissing and grinding against each other. At that point, you can tell she's into you. That's a good point to check in. If you can see she's nervous, reassure her that she doesn't need to do anything she doesn't want to do. Take the pressure off by keeping it relaxed and casual, and saying something like, "Let's take our time and enjoy tonight."

This section wouldn't be complete without some comment on sexually transmitted diseases (STDs) and unwanted pregnancies. I'm not here to wag a finger at you and tell you to use a condom, but equally, you may not know all that much about a woman's sexual history the first couple of times you're with her.

I don't find sex with a condom as pleasurable as without, so I sometimes add a drop of lube inside the condom. If you do this, use a high-quality water-based lubricant. When I go down on a woman who I don't know that well, I sometimes use a dental dam, which is a sheet of clear plastic, to prevent body fluids mingling. It's basically a condom for eating a woman out. One solution, which I sometimes use when I'm at a sex party, is to cut a condom in half and put that over a woman's genitals. It doesn't taste great, but it's better than getting an STD. Use your common sense and don't go down on someone whose pussy looks inflamed, discolored, or smells off.

People say that using a condom can be awkward to bring into the conversation. Yeah, it can be, but it's a lot less awkward than potentially catching an STD and having to tell every chick you're with that you've got something.

I want to share some hard truths from my own life here. I've had four pregnancy scares in my life. One of them happened when I was still working as a carpenter, struggling financially. When I found out she was pregnant, I was gutted. I blamed her. I started to suspect that she had gotten pregnant on purpose.

I didn't think she would have the baby, but she decided she wanted it. I was a young guy who didn't feel ready to be a father. She was on the pill, which was supposed to be 97 percent effective, and I was cumming inside her like a machine, thinking I was invincible. It turns out 97 percent isn't 100 percent. Nowadays, I only cum inside a woman if I want to make a baby. There are so many variables with the pill. Is a woman taking it consistently? Is she healthy? What's her diet like? I wish I'd known all this at the time.

For a couple of months, we argued a lot about what the baby meant for our relationship, with me blaming her and her fighting back. Eventually, I accepted that I was going to be a father. I let go of my resentment and came to terms with the situation. Hard as it was, I gave her my full support. I even started to get excited about being a dad. We agreed to go to the twelve-week scan together, to find out whether the baby was a boy or a girl. Although I lacked the emotional maturity to deal with it well, I did my best to be supportive.

It was a stressful time. I was working sixty hours a week for a boss I hated, making about $400 AUD ($304 USD) a week. I was living at my girlfriend's house, knowing I would be a dad soon, but unable to discuss it with anyone. I was also training for a boxing fight. The day before the three-month scan, I got a call telling me she had left work early because she was bleeding everywhere. I was at boxing, and when I checked my phone, I had dozens of missed calls. All her girlfriends were calling me, trying to get hold of me. By the time I got the message, she was at the hospital and had miscarried.

I share this because a lot of guys think, "It'll never happen to me." If you're not careful, it can. I know from experience. If you're still thinking, "It won't happen to me," go hang out at an abortion clinic and talk to some chicks who have experienced a termination. It can happen, and when it does, it's terrible for everyone involved.

Something else I've learned from experience is how easy it is to contract an STD. I've had gonorrhea, chlamydia (twice), and herpes. Gonorrhea and chlamydia are reasonably easy to treat, but herpes is not just for Christmas, it's for life. I have to have that conversation every time I'm with someone new, even if I don't have an outbreak at the time.

Although herpes is more common than you might think, it is manageable. But it's better not to get it. I'm not condemning you if you choose to have unprotected sex, but I want you to understand the risks.

AFTERCARE

Aftercare is an important part of leaving her better and wetter. After sex, a lot of guys roll over and go to sleep, or they switch on Netflix and get lost in a TV series. It's fun to cuddle a while and relive the experience by taking a sex survey. Ask her what she liked and highlight the beautiful moments you shared. Share your favorite experiences and discuss what you'd like to do next time. Even if you're exhausted, do this before falling asleep.

Do the things you'd like someone to do for you—for example, getting her a glass of water. If you've got something sweet like ice cream to snack on, dig it out of the freezer and offer to share it with her. You may want to invite her to stay over and get her breakfast the next day, but if not, make sure she gets home safely. Walk her downstairs, put her in a cab, or pay for her Uber. Whatever suits your circumstances.

These are little ways of communicating that you respect her and like her as a person, and that you're not simply using her for sex. Send her an appreciative message to let her know you enjoyed seeing her and—if you want to—that you'd like to see her again. A woman who has opened up deeply during sex may come back to earth and feel insecure. It's vulnerable to show herself so deeply. Take care of her and reassure her that everything's okay.

Don't underestimate the power of the material in this book. A recent client had a few sexual experiences with a woman he met in Bali. After a while, he decided he didn't want to see her again. Although he broke things off respectfully, the woman couldn't speak to him for four months. Eventually they ran into each other at a café, where she explained that the experiences had been so great that she found it hard to get over him.

THE LIFE CYCLE CONNECTION

I was very reluctant to put this exercise and the next one in the book, because they're so powerful and can be easily misused. Usually, I only teach them behind closed doors to clients I trust. Please, use them ethically.

When you're serious about a woman, an incredible way to deepen the connection is to talk about what you'll do together. This is like catnip to women, so be ethical. Calibrate it to what you truly want. Don't start talking about marriage and kids and a dog with a woman you only want to spend one night with.

That said, have fun with it. When you're with a lover, you can talk about what you want to do together. If the relationship evolves into something more serious, judge the life cycle connection according to how you're feeling. It's a beautiful way to develop a connection.

Exercise:
Create a Life Cycle Connection

When you're ready, sit down together and chat about the life cycle connection. The timeline of your relationship extends into the past as well as the future. Talk about who you both were before you met, and your shared past up to this point. Remind each other how you first met, and discuss your first experiences together, right up to the present day. This is a great way to reminisce about what first drew you together.

You can even take it back further. Ask her where she was born, what she remembers of her early life, important experiences in childhood. Give her time and space to show the stories that have shaped her—both light and dark.

Once you've set the scene, you can move the timeline into the future. What are your individual future goals? What goals do you share? How do you fit into each other's lives? What experiences do you want to have together? How do you see your relationship developing? Will you live together? Get married? Have kids? How will your sex life together evolve and flourish over the years?

Again, this is incredibly powerful. It will form a deep, profound bond. So, use it with care.

THE FANTASY REALITY

Another version of the life cycle connection is the fantasy reality. Again, this is a killer. When you do this, you'll have women eating out of your hand. The emotional mind can't tell the difference between fantasy and reality, so these fantasies will feel very real. Don't fuck with the women in your life. Calibrate it to match your intentions.

In the fantasy reality, you pick a scenario and imagine together how you got there. Introduce it by saying, "Let's play a game." For example, you can imagine where you'll be together in ten years' time, and how you will get there. You can then extend the timeline twenty or thirty years into the future, right up until death. This is an opportunity for her to use her imagination and create a story about how you get from where you are now to an imagined future. All the crazy shit you do, all the dreams and desires you fulfill together. Dive into detail, including everything from nicknames and pet names to inside jokes. How can you build a world together, in which each of the stories you tell builds another piece of your shared reality?

Maybe you travel to an exotic location together and enjoy crazy, risky adventures. You get the idea. When you play this game, you'll get an incredible insight into her fantasies. You can dive into the details. What will she wear on your wedding day? What will her father say when he gives her away? Who will the bridesmaids be? What happens after the wedding? What will you call your kids? Your pets? What will the sex be like when you're old and wrinkly? How will you die? What will be the last words you speak to each other (like *The Notebook*)?

Talk about where your lives will take you individually, and how you'll fit into each other's lives. Describe the joint creation you will build together.

You can imagine how powerful this exercise is, especially when she's telling you about it and becoming animated as she tells you about your lives together. She's literally envisioning marrying you and spending her life with you. That's why you should only use it with a woman you're really into.

At the other end of the spectrum, keep it smaller. Let's say you're on a first date and things are going well. Try, "Hey, imagine a crazy adventure that you would want to have with me." What will the setting be? What will we do? Even at this scale, it's an insane window into the mind of a woman. Take it to whatever level is right for you and the woman you're with.

THANK-YOU SEX

When you get all of this right, you'll blow a woman's mind. That's when you may notice that girls start to look at you with puppy-dog eyes and want to please you as much as you please them. It's a phenomenon I call thank-you sex.

Thank-you sex isn't about performing any specific moves or practices. It's more about an attitude. It's sex with a grateful woman who wants to celebrate how much she enjoys connecting with you. She may show you her appreciation in any number of ways, from kisses and cuddles to weekends away to frequent blow jobs. The point here is that the cultural stereotype is that men always want to have sex, while women lack libido and don't want it as much. So wrong.

When you become the kind of man described in these pages, you won't have that problem. She will thank you for giving her incredible experiences and brag to her friends about how you treat her inside and outside the bedroom. You'll probably notice those friends looking at you differently. We've even heard stories of women flying our clients around the world just so they could experience round two.

Oh, and if you'd like to get her obsessed with giving you head, check out the training on exactly that at sexualquantumleap. com/resources.

THE DARK SIDE OF BEING THE BEST SHE EVER HAD

It's not all thank-you sex, however. There is a dark side to being amazing in bed. Like hot women who everyone wants, you'll find that you're in great demand. You'll likely need to make some hard choices about how you spend your time.

Women may playfully tell you that they hate you because you've ruined them for other men, or they may genuinely be angry with you because you're not willing to give them the attention they want. The challenges that come with being highly attractive are different from the challenges that come with lacking confidence and experience, but they're no less real. You'll go from having trouble getting women to stay around to having them crave your cock and tell you you're the best they ever had.

If you're seeing multiple women, you'll need to handle their expectations. You may need to gently tell some women that you're no longer available to spend time with them. These are the challenges that come with being in demand.

Of course, you're a cool guy with a good heart, so you're not going to fuck with the women in your life. You're not going to use this material to coerce, manipulate, or otherwise hurt women you connect with. Instead, you're going to treat women with respect, share great experiences with them, and handle their emotions kindly. When you blow a woman's mind, she'll want to see you again. She might feel hurt and disappointed if you don't want to, because she'll never have that experience again.

RYKO'S STORY: PART II

In his heart, Ryko craved a deep connection with one partner. At the retreat, he did an exercise where he walked toward the model, Kim, and held eye contact with her.

Every time we do this exercise, someone breaks down. It's incredible how even the toughest guys feel their armor falling away. For Ryko, the effect was profound. As he walked toward the model, he broke down and began to cry. Soon, he was bawling his eyes out. I was crying with him. The whole room was crying. Finally, he stopped, looked at the model, looked at me, and said, "I can finally love again." Still makes me cry when I think about it.

Two weeks later, Ryko met a woman and fell in love. The pain he was carrying around with him for thirty years faded away, and he was capable of being present and connecting deeply. He told me that the sex is the deepest, most intimate experience of his life, and that the connection only gets better with time. For Ryko, the craziest sexual experience of all is looking into his partner's eyes, telling her how much he cares about her, and making love to her.

CONCLUSION

I did an event in Melbourne where I gave a talk and gave away $500 worth of sex toys. I felt like Santa Claus.

At the start of the talk, I was mucking around with an SQL team member, doing some Brazilian Jiu-Jitsu (BJJ). Not the most professional image to present, but fuck it. I don't know a lot about BJJ, but I was having fun, wrestling and rolling around on the floor. Another guy walked in and saw us—unbeknownst to me, he was a high level BJJ master. I was worried that he'd be put off, but instead he was instantly at ease. He thought it was cool.

The guy's name was Dainis. I gave a two-hour talk and he stayed around at the end to chat. He bought a toy called the Wand—which, by the way, I highly recommend—and asked if he could practice a bit on the doll. I wound up chatting with him for about ten minutes and giving him a demonstration. He went home, did what I taught him, and blew a woman's mind. "Damn," he thought. "If that was the free seminar, bring on the retreat."

Dainis was in the middle of reinventing himself. He was a successful businessman who made a lot of money, but then he lost it all. He was rebuilding, figuring out who he was without all his wealth. Despite this big shift in his circumstances, Dainis was a cool, fun-loving guy. He sold three of his friends on coming to the retreat, just on the strength of telling them about his experiences and our chat. In particular, he brought his best buddy, G-Dog.

Walking in, Dainis was a brash, confident guy. His reversal of fortune hadn't damaged his self-esteem in the bedroom. He had big ideas about getting into some crazy sexual situations, and he wanted to bring G-Dog along for the ride. G-Dog wasn't so into it. He was a little older and more interested in finding a life partner he could be with. Nonetheless, G-Dog wanted to support Dainis. If that meant going to a few sex parties, he was willing to give it a try.

I wanted Dainis to have whatever experiences he really wanted, but I got a sense that he wasn't as into the crazy stuff as he claimed. There was something about the way he talked about his desires that gave me the impression he was saying what he thought he *should* want, rather than what he actually wanted.

With eight years of BJJ training, and about the same amount of time doing Tae Kwon Do, Dainis was a walking weapon. He could kill a guy with his bare hands. But he was so focused on controlling his strength that he didn't know how to express himself in an animalistic way. He was scared of his own power. He was also scared of doing anything he felt was degrading to women. He told me about taking a chick home who wanted him to spit in her mouth and slap her face. He felt weird about it. "I love my mom and I love women," he told me. "I didn't want to disrespect her." This was despite the fact that she specifically requested all of that, and more.

To break down his conditioning, I got in his face and yelled that women want to feel his power. I could see something clicked and he let go. Straight after that, we went into an exercise about envisioning a perfect partner, and he lost it. He finally let go of fearing his power and burst into tears.

After years of holding back his power and strength, Dainis felt like he could express his primal emotions without being controlled by them. That freed him up to go wild, and also to discover deep connections.

Despite a few attempts to get G-Dog interested in crazy nights, G-Dog got clear that he didn't want to play that game. Dainis finished the retreat and went home to live out all his crazy fantasies—then called me to tell me about them. He really took it up a few notches. But then, once Dainis got it out of his system, he wound up connecting deeply with G-Dog's sister. They fell in love and developed an intimate, meaningful sexual relationship.

Behind the brashness and the desire for crazy times, Dainis is a gentle, amazing guy who craved a loving, deep connection with someone who he felt got him. A lot of what he originally wanted was about seeking external validation after losing so much money. Once he worked through that, it became clear that his deeper desire was to enjoy a profound connection with one woman.

BE GENUINELY ALPHA

A few final thoughts on becoming a man who will attract incredible women and share amazing experiences. There's a lot of bullshit written about how to be an alpha male. Being alpha isn't about being domineering and hypermasculine. A true alpha male tries to lift people up and make them better. There are four big areas I think men need to focus on to become truly alpha: health, wealth, relationships, and spirituality.

Your health is about how well you take care of yourself. I'm not saying you need to be a model, but do you eat well? Do you get enough rest and exercise? Is your body functioning and mobile, so that you have the energy to be active in the bedroom? Personally, I love yoga, calisthenics, swimming, wakeboarding, and trekking epic mountains.

Similarly, financial success isn't defined by a number in your bank account. It isn't necessarily about having millions of dollars. It's about your relationship with money. Find something you're inspired to teach the world and turn it into a business. If you're doing a job you hate and feel like life's constantly getting you down, you're not going to feel wealthy. On the other hand, if you love your work, you may feel wealthy even if you're not making millions.

Set your money up so that it works for you, paying you a monthly salary and allowing you to live the life you want to live, spending time with people who inspire you and having epic sex. Read books and attend seminars on money, investing, and business. A fundamental principle is paying yourself first, which means putting a set portion of your income aside every month, and raising it by 10 percent every three months. These are the things that contribute to a sense of wealth. Success isn't necessarily about having loads of money. It's about how you spend your time. Nonetheless, sex definitely feels better when I know I have money in the bank. If you're stressed about money, you'll be stuck at the bottom of Maslow's Hierarchy of Needs, focused on survival. That will definitely hinder your sexual pleasure and your capacity to be present in the bedroom. To me, true wealth and success come from having enough money to do what I want, when I want, with whom I want, for as long as I want.

To really shift your mindset around money, try fucking on money. Take a good chunk of cash out of your bank account and fuck on money. Get dressed up, then come back to your place, throw the money in the air so that it lands on the bed, and get to it. Set up a role-play where the woman pretends to be a stripper or a sex worker. Step into your power as a rich sex god. You truly can have it all—money, women, and a deep sense of purpose. Whenever I've done this with women, they get so horny. It's an amazing way to create positive associations between money and sex, two things that people often have negative associations with. It goes without saying that you should only do this with a chick you trust!

I'll never forget something my mum once told me: "People come into your life for a reason, a season, or a lifetime." Relationships with the most important people in your life are such a key component of happiness. The quality of your life is defined by the quality of your relationships. How well do you connect with your parents, siblings, and friends? Are you surrounded by a community of people who lift you up? Mama Kamakshi, my Reiki mentor, made me write out the following affirmation hundreds of times: "I'm happy and grateful now that I am always surrounded by people who understand me, care for me, and support me. I now accept love care and nourishment." These words have become true and will stay with me for the rest of my life.

As I define it, spirituality isn't about speaking Sanskrit, wearing a robe, or changing your name to Wood Stump. It's about being in tune with a mission bigger than yourself and living from your soul's calling. I don't care whether you're openly religious, but I do think it's essential for every guy to have a sense of a greater purpose in life. When I wake up in the morning, I spend time with people I love, doing things that I love. That's my idea of a spiritual life.

You might not see Warren Buffett as a spiritual man, but I do. He's a man on a mission who loves what he does. He seems to have found his soul's calling when he started investing at the age of ten, and he hasn't stopped since. He is lit up and inspired by what he does. If you're living your highest values and feeling a sense of inspiration, that is your spiritual path. John Demartini refers to this as your *telos*; your chief aim, living from your highest values. When you follow your *telos*, you will feel alive, like you're doing what you were put on this planet to do, and your life will keep getting better and better. This is my idea of a true spiritual path. Women will feel it when you're aligned with your *telos*. When you love what you do, it'll shine out of you. It's a damn attractive quality.

THE BITCH ACRONYM

If you want to keep a woman around, there are five essential character traits you need to model: backbone, integrity, tenacity, character, and humility. Backbone is what it takes to show up vulnerably, but to also be strong when your strength is called upon. A man with backbone expresses and maintains boundaries when he needs to. He doesn't take shit.

Integrity means that you say what you mean, and you mean what you say. Your word is your bond, and you do what it takes to protect the value of your words. Tenacity comes from the drive and determination to make things happen, and a refusal to give up. How do you bounce back when things don't go your way?

When you have character, you're living with the heart of a lion. You're inspired, and you value meaning in life over convenience. To quote Mahatma Gandhi, your aim is to "be the change you wish to see in the world."

Another great Gandhi quote is, "First they ignore you, then they laugh at you, then they fight you, then you win." When you stick your head over the wall, it will take a while for people to even notice. Then, you'll likely attract some ridicule and resistance before finally becoming known and accepted. That's how Sexual Quantum Leap became the number one school for sexual education.

Finally, a humble guy knows that there are limits to his knowledge. He's willing to accept those limits, learn from what life throws at him, and use the experience to become a better man.

You may already have realized that those traits add up to an acronym: BITCH. Which is ironic, because you won't be anyone's bitch if you make these qualities central to your life.

GREAT SEX IS...

Throughout this book, I've offered up loads of different ideas, concepts, and techniques. Ultimately, though, perhaps the biggest lesson is that great sex doesn't follow the rules. It's continuously surprising; sometimes we don't even know what we want.

This is why it's so important to realize that you're not going to get it right or perfect every time. We're not robots; we're not machines. Sometimes the perfection lies in the imperfection. Sex doesn't have to be a certain way. It's a beautiful, mysterious dance.

Whenever I meet someone new, I try to clear my mind of what I think it'll be like. I become like an excited kid at Christmas, eager to unwrap this new person and learn about their body, mind, and soul. For me, that's the excitement of sex. I never know what experiences are waiting for me.

Living out your fantasies is great, but if you are constantly trying to perform instead of being present, you'll inevitably be disappointed when it isn't as great in real life as it is in your head. You'll shut down the pleasure of connection and never truly experience the person in front of you.

Constraining yourself and your partner is the opposite of great sex. That's why it's so important to give yourself the freedom to explore what you want to explore, to express yourself through breath, sound, movement, and vocal expression, and to be open to what your partner likes.

Sexuality shifts constantly. As you mature, your tastes will change. You may find that you want more crazy experiences, or you may prefer to deepen a connection with one person. The only constant in life is change, so you might as well be present to the changing moods of your sexuality. What you like or how you like it might change. Ask yourself what you want and need. Dive into your sexuality and discover what fulfills you. Keep checking in with yourself and discerning what you want to try.

The more present you are to what's going on in the moment, the more you'll be able to relax. That makes it more likely you'll be able to get out of your head and into your body. Don't beat yourself up over performance. That will only take you into your anxieties and, ironically, make it harder to enjoy the experience.

Whatever's going on for you, it's okay. If you do find it hard to express your sexuality, cum too quickly, or struggle to get it up, remember that you're not broken. There's nothing wrong with you. Whatever level you're at, there will always be new challenges. A couple years from now, you may be wondering how to satisfy two women at once.

Anything you're struggling with can be addressed. When you empower yourself sexually, you can have the sex life you desire and deserve. Don't let anyone tell you what's right or wrong for you. Find out for yourself. If there's one message I want you to take from this book, it's that you have complete permission to develop a sexual life that's right for you. Think for yourself and question everything you read in these pages. Test out everything you've learned and let the results speak for themselves.

I hope the stories you've read in these pages have already given you permission to create the sex life you want. If not, let me reiterate: you don't know what's possible until you try. Sex is like any other area of your life. If you want to be good in business, or get ripped at the gym, you need to put in time and effort. Sex is no different. Change won't happen overnight, but it will happen if you consistently put your attention on your sexuality.

Is it worth it? That's up to you. What's the alternative? A mediocre sex life for the rest of your days? A sexless marriage? Every one of the stories in these pages is about a man just like you who took a chance on changing this area of his life. With dedication and commitment, they all got to a place they couldn't have imagined. Now it's your turn to take the leap.

BEST SHE EVER HAD

What's it worth to you to hear women saying, "Wow, that was amazing"? What's it worth to have women eager to see you again, telling their friends about the great experiences you had together?

It's totally possible. Women bringing their girlfriends to meet you. Or, if you're in a committed relationship, your wife wanting sex more often. A sense of invigoration and confidence. "I've never had a man touch me like that." "How do you know my body so well?" When you hear words like these coming out of a woman's mouth, it feels amazing. (Your partner saying thank you for being in my life, I appreciate you so much.)

Just remember to stay present and enjoy each moment and let the beauty of your sexual journey consistently unfold. As Paige Toon beautifully said, "Don't wait for the storm to pass, learn to dance in the rain."

WHAT NEXT?

If you've got value from reading this book, I highly recommend that you visit sexualquantumleap.com/resources. The material you'll find there will take you to the next level. Start by watching the exclusive training that comes at the top of the page. Then, explore the rest of the resources you'll find on that page. We've already helped thousands of men become the best she ever had, and we want you to be the next.

If you're ready to play full out, go to sexualquantumleap.com/apply and fill out the form you find there. This is a short application for an exploratory call to find out whether we're a good fit to work together.

Every man deserves a true sexual education so he can feel free and satisfied in this area of his life. Let's throw off the shackles of sexual mediocrity together and spread the messages in this book far and wide.

ACKNOWLEDGMENTS

Granny: Thank you for being the rock in the family and my life. You are so kind, wise, and caring. Thank you for supporting me through everything. I love you very much.

Dad: Thank you for instilling such a strong work ethic, entrepreneurial spirit, and never-say-die attitude in me. Thank you for teaching me about integrity and hard work. Thank you for keeping me level-headed, when at times I can be a crazy whirlwind.

Mum: When I was growing up, my mum used to say to me, "I don't care what you do. I don't care if you work as a garbage man, as long as you are happy." I love you dearly, mother!

Frank (Stepdad): Frank, I can't thank you enough for encouraging me to keep pursuing my goals. You instilled in me a sense of hope and a willingness to think big.

Daniel Mioch: Thank you for being my little brother and my biggest supporter since day one. Thank you for all the encouragement and for pushing me to be the man I am today.

Thank you for supporting me through some of the hardest times in my life. I'll never forget the time you lent me $200 so I could rent a car and go to a shitty job, all so I could keep pursuing a bigger vision. We did it, man. I really couldn't have done it without you.

Jessica Mioch: I love you. I have nothing more to say.

Steve Resic and Family: My dearest childhood friend. Your family adopted me as their own and I am forever grateful. I'll never forget rocking up to your house at the age of seventeen, saying I had lost my virginity, and all the experiences we have had together since! Thank you for seeing me through everything. I love you so much, brother.

Jamie Tomic: You are like family to me and the backbone of this company. Thank you for everything you do for me, personally and professionally. SQL wouldn't be close to where it is today without you.

Sim (Black Mamba): Thank you for being my best friend and support for close to ten years. Thank you for your love and friendship, and for being with me through all these crazy times. We are changing the world, brother, one person at a time. Thank you for being right by my side.

James Hepburn: Thank you for kicking me in the ass in the early days of SQL. Thank you for telling me how much it changed your life and pounding in the message that I had to get this message out into the world. Thank you for your being a good mate and for all the support you have given SQL.

ACKNOWLEDGMENTS

Magida Ezzat: Thank you for constantly encouraging me to pursue my mission in the world, and for giving your loving female perspective—not to mention coming up with the name Sexual Quantum Leap while we were housemates talking shit in the kitchen.

Pierre De Sousa: Thank you for yelling at me and telling me to stop fucking around and teach sex full-time, and also for being by my side on SQL's first international tour.

Shae Matthews: Thank you for being my first mentor on sexuality, spirituality, and masculinity. You really helped lay the foundations of the man I am today and the work I share with the world. Your love, care, humility, and willingness to serve humanity is forever admirable.

Dominic (The Dom): Thank you for showing me what it means to be a dominant man and introducing me to the endless possibilities of sexuality. Thank you for my early education in sexuality, spirituality, and life.

Red: Thank you for taking me under your wing and teaching me so much about female sexuality and what women actually want in the bedroom, including the infamous "pussy massage" and the secrets of eating pussy. You are such a beautiful woman with a big heart.

Tao Semko: You are such a profound mentor in my spiritual and sexual life. You have really inspired me to learn what it means to be a man, and to show up with love and integrity in this world. I am forever grateful.

Lawrence Petruzzelli: Thank you for believing in me and supporting me since day one. SQL wouldn't be close to where it is without you. You always believed in me when no one else did, man. I will never forget that.

Ron Malhotra: Thank you for seeing something in me and taking me under your wing from day one, when I had hardly any money. Thank you for seeing the man I was and the impact I wanted to make in the world. Thank you for helping me set a global vision for SQL.

Stuart Hallam: Thank you, brother, for supporting my personal development and the growth of SQL in the early days, and for encouraging me to take SQL out into the world. Also, thank you for being there at some of the hardest times in my life and guiding me through them, and for all you have taught me about sexuality.

Caleb Lesa: You have helped me see the code of life and relationships. Thank you for being an outstanding friend and mentor, and for supporting me in developing healthy relationships with everyone, most importantly myself.

Mama Kamakshi: Thank you for being my Reiki master, spiritual teacher, and Indian mama. Thank you for caring for me like your son, teaching me so much about Indian culture and, most importantly, my internal world.

Dr. John Demartini: Thank you for inspiring me to inspire the world, and to follow my *telos*. Thank you for teaching me the laws of the universe and being such a powerful mentor.

All the Women: To all the women I have been with and haven't been with, thank you for humbling me and teaching me how to be a better man and a better lover. Thank you, too, for all the beautiful messages about the work SQL is doing.

Scribe: To the amazing team at Scribe, especially my kick-ass editor, Big Dong Rob Wolf Petersen, and my wonderful publishing manager, Mikey Kershisnik. This book seriously wouldn't have been completed without you. I appreciate your guidance and support throughout the whole book publishing process.

The SQL Team: To all the people who have contributed to SQL in the past, present, and future. The reason we are here today is because of you. Thank you for believing in the vision and mission of the company, showing up every single day, and giving it your all. I see you all as family, and I appreciate everything you do, have done, and will do in the future.

All SQL Clients, Past, Present, and Future: You're the reason we do what we do. Our goal is to serve you. Thank you for trusting us.

You: Finally, a big thank you, to *you*, for reading this book all the way to the acknowledgements. Thank you for having the courage to invest in your sexual education, and the willingness to go to places most people never dare. This is how I know you'll live the kind of life most people never even dream of, and enjoy the wildest sexual adventures you can imagine.

CPSIA information can be obtained
at www.ICGtesting.com
Printed in the USA
BVHW031250080322
630893BV00006B/123